AGELESS
Pilates

Here's what Experts <u>and</u> Everyday People are saying about

AGELESS
Pilates

"I love the Ageless Pilates System as it gives you new tools to learn Pilates. As an instructor of the technique for 30 years, I find it's so important for clients to have effective ways of understanding the method."
- Michael King, International Pilates presenter, author of 10 Pilates books

Christine's **deep understanding of the body makes her a gift** *to both brand new students and those who have been working with their bodies for years.*
- Meghan P., Ageless Pilates client

"The ABC's of Ageless Pilates give you **a safe and effective workout** *that can be easily applied to daily life, allowing you walk taller and move freely."*
- Keri Cawthorne, Owner of Iron Mountain Movement, British Columbia, Canada

She will help you to discover the capabilities you never knew you had.
- Saundra L., Ageless Pilates client

"Ageless Pilates is **a terrific book** *that meets the needs of the many in an easy formula, everyone can use every day!"*
- Stacy A. Darkis Pilates Instructor & Breast Cancer Exercise Specialist
Studio 59 Pilates - Westbrook, Maine

"Ageless Pilates has **fantastic images and cues for correct alignment**. *This is a great book to guide you into beginning your exercise program with an emphasis on the foundations of the Pilates method."*
- Sherri Betz, PT, author of The Osteoporosis Exercise Book
and Owner of Thera Pilates Physical Therapy Studio, Santa Cruz, CA

The transformation of my body over the past year is nothing short of amazing.
- Susan S., Ageless Pilates client

AGELESS
Pilates

*The Secret to Moving Comfortably, Easily and Pain-free
for the Rest of Your Life*

Christine Binnendyk

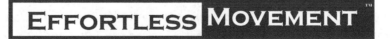

PORTLAND, OREGON

ISBN 978-0-9823170-0-6

Library of Congress Cataloging-in-Publication Data available

10 9 8 7 6 5 4 3 2 1

The information in this book is educational purposes only. It is not intended to replace the advice of a physician or medical practitioner. Please see your health care provider before beginning any new health program.

CONTENTS

Introduction 6

A note from Christine ■ About Ageless Pilates ■ Four Golden Rules ■ How to Use this Book ■ What to Wear ■ What Else will You Need

Chapter 1 ~ The ABC's 12

Begin at the Center ■ Create Your Anchor Points ■ Draw Your Box ■ Balance Your Teacup ■ Place Your Shoulders ■ Stack & Lengthen ■ Key Positions

Chapter 2 ~ Building Blocks 28

Lesson 1: Spine Warm-up ■ Lesson 2: Pelvis Warm-up ■ Lesson 3: Shoulder Warm-Up Lesson 4: Leg & Hip Warm-up ■ Workout 1: Building Blocks ■ Workout 2: Starfish

Chapter 3 ~ Matwork Basics 58

Lesson 5: Leg & Hip Moves ■ Lesson 6: Balancing Abdominals ■ Lesson 7: Shoulder Placement ■ Lesson 8: Tabletop Reach ■ Lesson 9: Lengthen the Spine ■ Workout 3: Matwork Basics ■ Workout 4: Long & Strong ■ Workout 5: Drawbridge

Chapter 4 ~ Your Powerhouse 88

Lesson 10: Lower Ab Focus ■ Lesson 11: Arm & Leg Coordination ■ Lesson 12: Double Duty ■ Lesson 13: Corset Cinch ■ Workout 6: Building the Powerhouse ■ Workout 7: Working the Powerhouse

Chapter 5 ~ Perfect Posture 112

Lesson 14: Side Stretch ■ Lesson 15: Chest Expansion ■ Lesson 16: Working the Wall ■ Lesson 17: Spine Extension ■ Workout 8: Lengthen and Strengthen ■ Workout 9: Feeling Tall

Chapter 6 ~ Balance Builders 134

Lesson 18: Kneeling Lunge ■ Lesson 19: Standing Balance ■ Lesson 20: Standing Lunge ■ Lesson 21: Wide Plies ■ Lesson 22: Narrow Plies ■ Workout 10: Building Balance ■ Workout 11: Growing Taller

Chapter 7 ~ Upper Body Mobility 152

Lesson 23: Mobile Shoulders ■ Lesson 24: Secret Weapon ■ Workout 12: Easy Shoulders, Easy Neck ■ Workout 13: Mobility Creates Strength

Chapter 8 ~ Workouts for Ailments 170

Workout 14: Low Back Tonic ■ Workout 15: Arthritis Relief ■ Workout 16: Bone Building ■ Workout 17: Seated Arm Work ■ Workout 18: Seated Leg Work

Index 180

A note from Christine

How would you love to spend your next free day? Playing bocce, golf or tennis? Strolling around your favorite city? Gardening in your yard? Chasing your children or grandchildren?

Sadly, many people assume that eventually they'll be forced to give up these activities. Maybe holding a toddler while cooking dinner has caused a permanent tweak in your low-back. One day, maybe a golf swing tweaks your back; or you stumble and take a fall; or you find that you can't get up after kneeling in the garden.

Many people expect that their body will give up on them over time.

When do you think that day might come, when you have to start giving up activities that you enjoy? 70? 60? 50? 40? Have you already started giving up activities?

Aging doesn't need to look this way. Life expectancy has improved dramatically in the last 50 years. You can start doing something right now to improve your quality of life to match your length of life.

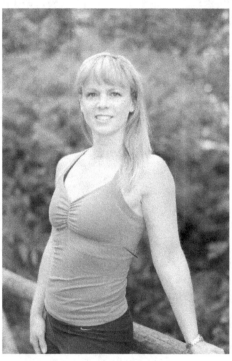

Age isn't what causes physical limitations. Improper body mechanics – mis-alignment, lost flexibility, and lack of strength – are the cause of many of today's chronic conditions. You can start improving all three areas of your body mechanics today, in just 15 minutes a day, using the **Ageless Pilates System**. A little bit of improvement each day will add up to a lifetime of enjoyable movement.

Fifteen minutes of Pilates a day can change everything you've ever thought about what you can count on your body to be able to do for the rest of your life. Let me say that again --- *For the Rest of Your Life.*

I work with people of all ages and in all stages of life. Almost everyone comes to me with aches and pains somewhere – back, neck and knee pain are the most common – and yet, I've never run into a person who couldn't ease their discomfort and improve their range of movement through the **Ageless Pilates system.**

Wherever you are in your life, you can find a program in this book that will help you. Find 15 minutes a day to transform your body. Make 15 minutes a day to transform your life for the better !

About Ageless Pilates

Joseph Pilates developed his system of **Contrology** in the early 1900's, incorporating more than 500 exercises that could be performed on a mat or on one of his specialized Pilates machines. He coined the term **Powerhouse** when he wrote about strengthening the center of the body to support all of your movements.

People from all walks of life — boxers, singers, dancers — flocked to his studio to learn his amazing system because it worked so well at re-aligning and re-building the body. Romana Kryzanowska, Joe's oldest living protégé, taught his classic method to me more than 10 years ago.

After working with thousands of clients, I've created the **Ageless Pilates System.** It marries together modern physical training expertise with the wisdom of Joseph Pilates' classical system.

Best of all, I've distilled the main concepts that will **transform your body mechanics and movement patterns** into three key areas. The **ABC's** of Ageless Pilates will give you a body that is strong and limber, comfortable and pain-free. Each 15-minute Lesson in this book will take you through the ABC's:

 Anchor Points give you stability. By learning your anchor points, you'll feel stable and confident in your movements.

 Body Geometry gives you structure. By learning how to arrange your body properly, you'll use your muscles to their best advantage.

 Comfort Options give you the flexibility to fine tune every exercise. You'll evaluate how your body feels in each position and in each movement pattern. I'll give tips on how to choose the best position and the most appropriate range of motion for you, in this moment.

I named this updated system **Ageless Pilates** to honor three of my Ageless heroes:

Joseph Pilates, a genius, who passed away in 1967 at age 87. He taught his fabulous system until the day he died, improving the lives of millions.

I can only hope to emulate these three innovators. They are tremendous examples of living a life that is not limited by age — they are Ageless. I'm hoping to inspire you to follow us to an Ageless Pilates way of life. Let's get going!

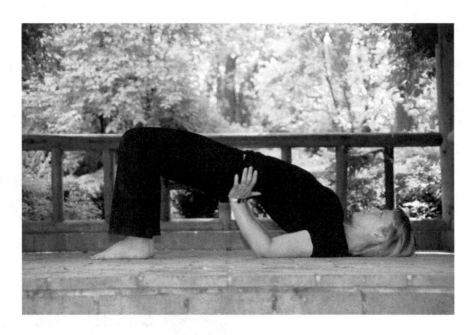

Jack Lalanne, a health icon to millions. My first memory of television is Jack performing his bicycle exercise as millions worked out along with him in the comfort of their own homes. He's still inspiring us in his 90's.

The amazing **Romana Kryzanowska,** who continues to travel, teach Pilates and live a full life in her 80's.

"you can start improving your body today"

The Four Golden Rules

Before we get deep into the Ageless Pilates system, let's look at the Four Golden Rules that will jumpstart your new movement program.

1. Move Everyday

Consistency is important in taking care of the one body that you get for this lifetime. We eat everyday, sleep everyday, and brush our teeth everyday. Your body needs to move everyday. Use this book as your guide for moving comfortably and without pain.

In this book, you now have a large menu of simple, **15-minute Ageless Pilates Lessons** and challenging, **30-minute Ageless Pilates Workouts**. Flip through the book to find something that piques your interest and get moving!

2. Remember to Breathe

We all feel so much better when we exhale. This book is your reminder to get back to the basics of using your breath to feel **relaxed**, **energized**, and **ready to go**. As you move through the chapters, you'll learn tips on Ageless Pilates breathing. Be sure to take a look at page 121 to read the benefits of creating nitric oxide as you breathe.

3. Listen to Your Body

Your body tells you what you need to know. This book is your guide to understanding what to do with the messages your body sends you.

This exercise makes my neck cranky means that it's time to adjust your **position**

THAT STRETCH FEELS GOOD means you've chosen an appropriate **range of motion**

I *can* do this movement pattern! means you've made a **good exercise choice** for today

Look at the **Body Geometry Tips** in each Movement Lesson; they'll help you decipher the messages that your body is sending out.

4. Always Balance Movement with Stability

Put quite simply, *when one body part moves, another body part stays still to anchor it.* This is the key to using the Ageless Pilates system to re-set your body for comfortable movement.

Notice the questions in each exercise; these are clues to heighten your awareness of stability and comfort. They'll help you decide if you need to adjust either your **position** or your **range of motion**. Study the **Anchor Points** in each Movement Lesson; they'll spell out how to create stability while you move.

How to Use this Book

Begin with the **ABC's chapter,** where you'll learn all about the key concepts behind the Ageless Pilates exercises — **Anchor Points**, **Body Geometry**, and **Comfort Options**.

The human body is an intelligent system. Once you've been introduced to these three concepts, you may notice your body responding with comfortable posture, loose and easy movement patterns, or a renewed sense of energy.

These are signs that your body has begun to choose more efficient patterns instead of the habits you've learned across your lifetime.

In Chapters 2-7, you'll add another layer to your patterns: movement.

Each chapter contains several **Lessons**, which take about 15 minutes the first few times you do them. Take your time, use the cues to find a way to make each movement comfortable.

Again, you are developing new patterns that will carry into your daily life. Some patterns will shift instantly, some require repetition and patience.

I love seeing that 'click' of recognition in my clients when **the body inhabits a new pattern** and the mind recognizes it. From that moment, the new pattern — whether it's how you naturally position your body, or how you move it — is yours to keep.

It's ok to work on several **Lessons** in a chapter, one right after the other, but don't feel the need to rush yourself. Your body needs some time to integrate each new pattern, and there is no telling exactly how long you'll need.

Once you've worked your way through all of the **15-minute Lessons** in an individual chapter, and you feel confident in the movements, go to the end of the chapter to find the **30-minute Workouts.** These workouts combine several movement patterns from the complete chapter.

Chapters 2 and 3 cover Building Blocks and Matwork Basics. You could do these exercises alone each day for the rest of your life, and find that you're able to do what you love during the day. You may not feel the need to add anything else.

> "We do not cease to play because we grow old
>
> We grow old because we cease to play"
> ~ George Bernard Shaw

Or, you may feel so energized that you choose to add more challenges or exercises that can help you address specific issues like **balance**, **posture**, or **flexibility**. Simply flip to those chapters and add on a **Lesson** or even a **Workout**.

Chapter 8 gives special notes for those managing **low back issues**, **arthritis**, and **dwindling bone density**. If you need to exercise while seated, you'll also find notes here.

Whether you spend 15, 30, 45 or 60 minutes is entirely up to you. You could sneak in a **Lesson** first thing in your day and maybe do a **Workout** later. **Whatever works for you is fine.** Set yourself up for success by choosing times that work for you, and making a commitment to **set these times aside every day.**

Many of my clients make their exercises a 'first thing in the morning' ritual and use them to get a jump start on their day.

Some people enjoy using their exercises as a little stress break at lunchtime or at the end of their workday. If another time of day works better for you, that's fine, but do make this commitment to yourself.

Over time, creating a daily habit will create a tremendous shift in your body.

What to Wear

While doing your Ageless Pilates exercises, it's best to wear lightweight clothing that allows you to comfortably stretch and move around. Avoid clothing that will be uncomfortable or distracting.

What Else will you need?

You can perform your Pilates exercises in a carpeted area, or on an exercise mat. Use care in selecting your padding for exercises. You don't want a squishy surface, but you do want any bony areas that come in contact to feel comfortable. Each person's body is different – one person may have backbones that are closer to the surface, another may have a sensitive tailbone, or front hipbones that protrude a bit. Make your choice based on your own comfort.

Items that you might find helpful to have in easy reach:

- Yoga strap or a soft belt or band
- Rolled up beach towel or a 6-8 inch soft ball
- Sturdy Chair
- 2 small water bottles or light hand weights

How to Breathe

In the beginning, I'm happy as long as my clients are breathing! So many people hold their breath when attempting something new, that I consider it a wonderful first step to just move and breathe at the same time.

As you become more comfortable with the positions and movements, you'll want to fine tune your breathing as well. When you exhale, do it completely. Really empty your lungs, so that your body is craving the next inhale. The trick is to do this with control. Synch up the exhale to take the exact amount of time as your movement. Make your next inhale synch up with the next movement. One inhale or exhale for each movement. Take your time when moving and breathing. If you breathe too quickly, you'll feel light-headed

As you become more confident, take care to exhale and inhale on the proper movements in each exercise. This takes quite a bit of concentration at first. **I know you can do it!**

"Do what you can, with what you have, where you are"
~ Teddy Roosevelt

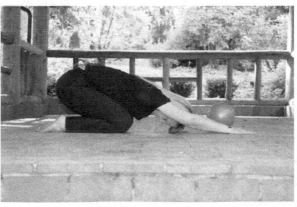

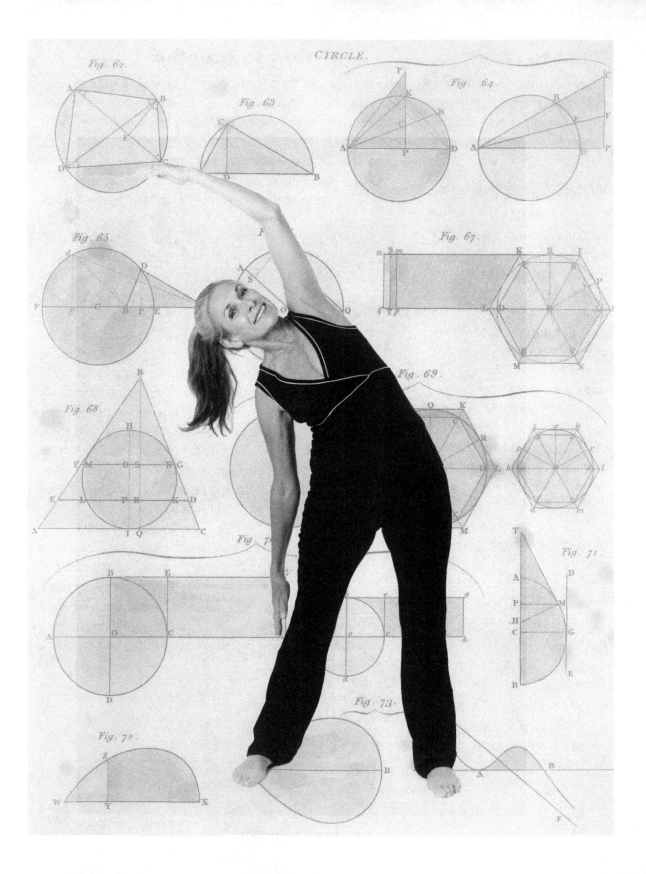

1

THE ABC'S

The **ABC's** are a system that will guide you in making good choices toward comfortable, pain-free movement.

When you're actively using your **Anchor Points, Body Geometry**, and **Comfort Options**, your skeleton is stacked up properly and your muscles are working efficiently. Movement feels easy and almost effortless. This is because your muscles are using just the right amount of energy and your joints are experiencing the least amount of wear and tear. Sounds good doesn't it?

The flip side of this is when your ABC's have gone off track. Maybe you sprained an ankle or tore a ligament in your knee, and your body began to compensate for the injury. Or maybe natural tendencies like slouching or hiking a hip up have become ingrained patterns. Any of these things can lead to poor positioning, and the one-two punch of overused muscles paired with atrophied muscles.

Your body doesn't know how to let go of these inefficient habits, until you introduce healthier patterns, like the ABC's. This system gives you the tools to make good choices for your movement patterns. **You'll know by the way you feel --- easy, effortless.**

BEGIN AT THE CENTER

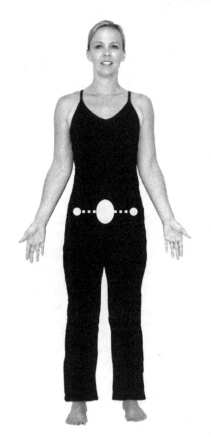

Where is the center of your body?

Draw an imaginary line from one hipbone to the other. We'll call this your **Baseline.** The center of this line is your **Center of Movement**.

■Place your fingertips on your hipbones. As you exhale, try to draw in this center point a bit. ■Try to initiate all movements and muscular effort from as close to this Center as possible.

Soon, you'll notice a wonderful shift in your Body Geometry. You'll find yourself re-distributing your weight and balancing your load more efficiently.

"almost magically, your body will re-align itself"

For women, the **Baseline** and **Center of Movement** correspond with our natural center of gravity. For men, their center of gravity — where the most muscle mass is found — is at the shoulders. This can mean it takes a little more 'mind over matter' for men to begin their movement from the Baseline. **No worries, you can do this.**

Body Geometry Tips are marked with this symbol

Body Geometry is all about putting your body in the best position for stability and movement. Find tips in these boxes to help you perfect your position. Look for them as you work through your Lessons. They'll give answers to common questions.

CREATE YOUR ANCHOR POINTS

Take a look at the balloons on the right. If they weren't **anchored** down with that little box, they'd float away with the ribbons dangling down.

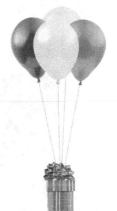

Imagine the balloons as your head, the ribbon as your body, and the box as.....you guessed it: your **Baseline,** which is also an **Anchor Point**. The body works more efficiently when it has strong anchors for each movement. They create a pivot point for the movements to originate from.

By creating Anchor Points, you'll be telling the body which muscles to use. ■**Notice:** when your anchor point is your Baseline, what muscles are connected right there? Your abdominals!

When the appropriate muscles take on the work for each movement in your life, the others muscles get a chance to recover. This new habit will mean less stress and less wear on your body.

Your most important **Anchor Points** are the **Baseline** and **Center of Movement.** If you're ever unsure of what to do, bring your focus back to the center of your body. I'll ask you to engage additional Anchor Points in each position. Sometimes this can feel like too many things to keep track of; **simply do what you can today, and check back over time**.

Try this: wave your hand and arm while moving your shoulder around. Yes, that was silly. And it wouldn't be an easy method for grabbing a can out of your cupboard. Now, try dropping your armpit low as you wave your hand and arm. Grabbing that can off the shelf now would be easy, wouldn't it? You just balanced your movement with a stable **Anchor Point.**

Anchor Points are marked with this symbol

Anchor Points are where you'll focus your muscular activity before you even start to move. They'll give you stability and they'll keep you safe throughout your movements. Look for these boxes as you work through your **Lessons**. Make sure you feel confident performing each movement while activating them, before you move on to your **Workouts** at the end of each chapter.

DRAW YOUR BOX

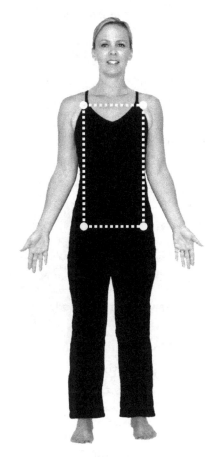

Shoulders

■Imagine a line from one shoulder to the other. ■**Notice** whether your shoulders are lined up with each other, or one shoulder rides higher than the other.

Imagine an Anchor Point at each Armpit

Gently draw the armpit toward your hip. ■**What just happened to your shoulders?** For many people, using an anchor point here will lower the shoulders and level them out.

Hips

■Try standing in front of a mirror and placing your pointer fingers on each hip bone while wrapping your hands around your hips. ■**Notice** whether your hands look level or one rides higher than the other. ■Can you level your hips if you try? As you continue your Body Geometry journey any discrepancies will lessen over time.

Completing the Box

■To complete The Box, imagine lines from right shoulder to right hip bone and left shoulder to left hip bone. Oftentimes, shifting a hip will affect the shoulder on the same side. ■Try standing with one hip cocked and notice the change in your shoulders in the mirror. Leave habits like this behind; they drain your energy and lead to discomfort.

Body Geometry Tip:
Re-think these Common Habits

- Do you carry a heavy bag on one shoulder rather than spreading the weight out?
- Do you use your shoulder to hold your phone, rather than using a hands free unit?
- Do you stand with all of your weight on one leg, rather than standing with your weight equally balanced?

BALANCE A TEACUP IN A TRIANGLE

Begin lying on your back with knees bent, feet hip width apart and flat on the floor.
■**Create a triangle** with your hands as I have in the photos. Place the heels of your hands on your hip bones. Point your fingers toward your pubic bone. ■In an ideal world, your triangle will be level with the floor and you'd be able to balance a teacup on it. Many trainers call this position **neutral pelvis;** I'll simply ask you to **balance your teacup.**

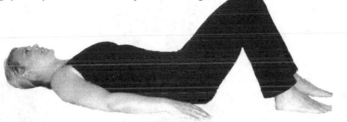

This position sets your muscles up to work efficiently. It also allows you to keep the natural curve of your low back. This **lumbar curve** protecting your discs and sacroiliac (SI) joint.

Create Anchor Points
at your Baseline and at the Soles of your Feet

- **Baseline;** scoop your belly in from hipbone to hipbone.
- **Soles of your Feet;** press these into the floor.

- **Notice what just happened!** For many people, activating your Anchor Points will level out the triangle.

Body Geometry Tip:

Notice Clues that your Position is not Ideal

■Does your triangle tilt to the left or right? ■Does your pubic bone drop or raise higher than your hip bones? ■Can you level out your triangle if you try? No worries if you find that you cannot level it out right now, we'll continue to work on this.

PLACE YOUR SHOULDERS

■With your hands on your head, shrug your shoulders up toward your earlobes. Feel your shoulder blades moving up your back. ■Lower your arms down, turning your palms forward. ■**Notice** how your shoulders have repositioned themselves far from your ears.

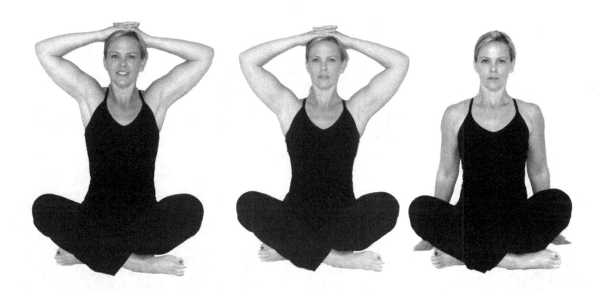

Create Your Anchor Points

■**Use your mind to create Anchor Points at your armpits and at the lowest tip of each shoulder blade.** ■Allow your Anchor Points to slide your shoulder blades down your back.

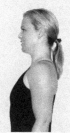

From the side, your shoulder should now line up with your ear.

When your shoulder blades sit well on the body, the movement of your arms feels as if it begins from your entire torso, giving you great stability. Suddenly, your arms feel almost weightless. This is a very different feeling than shortening the neck muscles to heave your arm upward. Placing your shoulders properly frees up your neck.

STACK AND LENGTHEN

Let's re-group by combining the first four pieces — Draw Your Box , Begin at the Center, Balance Your Teacup, Place Your Shoulders — into a **Stack.** The body is always strongest when your joints are stacked. Then, we'll take the **Stack** and **Lengthen** it.

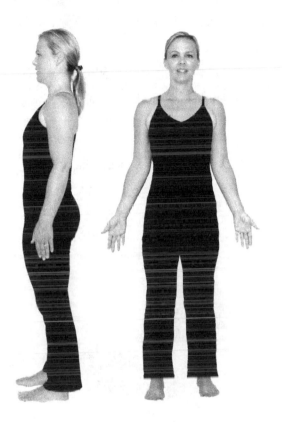

The Stack

Stand tall, and let's do a body scan:

■**Check your Box** Are your shoulders and hips level? Are the vertical line of the box even?

■**Begin at the Center** If you draw in hipbone to hipbone, can you stand a bit taller?

■**Balance your Teacup** Is your triangle level, or is it slightly tilted?

■**Place your Shoulders** Are your shoulder blades sliding comfortably down your back? Do you have plenty of space between your earlobe and your shoulder?

Why is this important? When your joints are stacked, the muscles are working in a balanced fashion. Each muscle does the job that it's meant to do, no more, no less. When you save energy based on your position, you can then spend it on movement.

The Lengthen

Imagine a string attached to the top your head. A puppeteer just lifted you up a smidgeon.

Notice what happened: ■Your neck became **long and loose**. ■Your collar bones are **floating gently** as your shoulder blades slide down the back. ■Your ribcage floats a bit above your hips, and they **each move independently.** ■Your hips, knees and ankles **feel loose.**

Key Positions are your starting point for each of the Ageless Pilates exercises. A quick glance at each picture may make these positions look simple. Simple isn't the same as easy though. Each position incorporates **Body Geometry, Anchor Points,** and **Comfort Options.** You're creating a strong structure and a system for transferring the energy that powers your movements in the upcoming exercises.

Comfort Options Are marked with this Symbol

Pilates is meant to be comfortable! Look for the Comfort Options marked with this symbol. They'll help you make choices that will take you out of the pain cycle.

■Choose your key position based on whether it is comfortable for you. ■Choose the size of your movement — your range of motion — based on whether it is comfortable for you. ■Advancing to the next position or the next bigger movement size is only advisable when you feel no pain or discomfort, **and** you're able to maintain your anchor points.

Try out each of the positions and anchor points as you read them. You may notice changes in how you hold your body immediately afterward and later in your day. **These are good signs that the Ageless Pilates system is carrying into your everyday life.**

KEY POSITION: Supine

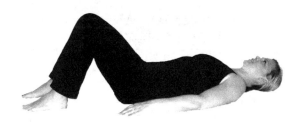

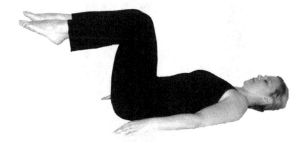

Supine/Knees Bent

■Lay on your back with your knees comfortably bent, feet flat on the floor. ■Line up your hip bones, knees and feet. ■Balance your teacup. ■Allow your low back to curve naturally. In other words, do not purposely flatten your back to the floor.

Supine/Legs Tabletop

■From Supine/Knees Bent Position, knit your ribcage together as if you were wearing a corset and float the knees directly over your hips. **We've removed an anchor point (your feet,) an added a new one: the ribcage.** ■Float your shins parallel to the floor. ■Your hip and knee joints should both be at a 90 degree angle. This will put you in a **stacked position,** which is an efficient starting point for movements.

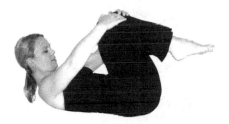
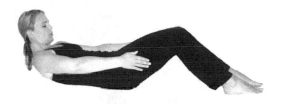

Mini Roll-up/Tucked

■From Supine/Knees Bent position, tuck your knees up to your chest. Grasp your knees when it becomes possible. ■Leading with your breast bone, lift your upper body forward and up a smidge.

■Your goal is to peel the top of your shoulder blade off your mat. ■**Use your upper abdominals to power the movement.**

Mini Roll-up/Feet Flat

■From Supine/Knees Bent position, reach your fingertips toward the sky. ■Think of your ribcage as a wheel. Roll the wheel forward. ■In other words: leading with your breast bone, curl your upper body toward your knees. Grasp your knees when it becomes possible.

■Your goal is to peel the top of your shoulder blade off your mat. ■**Use your upper abdominals to power the movement.**

Anchor Points for Supine Positions

Knees Bent
- **Baseline;** scoop in from hipbone to hipbone.
- **Seat:** squeeze your bottom.
- **Soles of your feet;** press these into the floor.

Legs Tabletop
- ■Baseline ■Seat *and...*
- **Ribcage;** knit the ribs inward, as if you were wearing a corset.

Mini Roll-up Tucked
- ■Baseline ■Seat ■Ribcage

Mini Roll-up Feet Flat
- ■Baseline ■Seat ■Soles of your feet

KEY POSITION: Seated

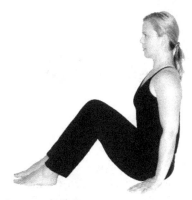

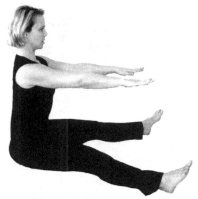

Seated/Knees Bent

■Sit on your mat as upright and tall as possible.
■Check your Stack: note how **my ear lines up over my shoulder joint,** and **my shoulder joint lines up over my hip joint.** ■Bend your knees so that you can place your feet flat on the floor.

Seated/Legs Extended

■Sit on your mat as upright and tall as possible. ■Extend and flatten your legs, gently pressing them into the mat to help **anchor** you. ■This may feel more difficult than sitting with your knees bent. Your legs are likely not accustomed to working in this position. Know that you'll become stronger over time.

Anchor Points **for Seated Positions**

Knees Bent

- **Baseline;** scoop in from hipbone to hipbone.
- **Seat;** squeeze your bottom.
- **Soles of your feet;** press these into the floor.
- **Ribcage;** knit the ribs inward, as if you were wearing a corset.

Legs Extended

■Baseline ■Seat *and...*
- **Legs;** gently press them into your mat.

Cross Legged

■Baseline ■Seat ■Ribcage

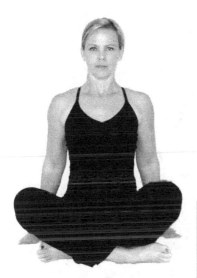

Seated/Cross Legged

■Since we've removed an anchor point — your legs/feet — sitting cross legged requires your abdominal muscles to work harder to balance you. ■It is not necessary to force this position. If it is uncomfortable for you., simply substitute another Seated position.

Body Geometry Tip:

Breathing while Corseting

■Draw your ribs together, as if you were putting on a tight dress. ■Breathe in through your nose. ■Notice: your upper back can expand to accommodate the air. You don't need to poof your belly out.

Body Geometry Tip: Check Your Stack

The Ageless Pilates system is highly adjustable; it allows you to choose positions and movements to fit your body's condition right at this moment.

Fine Tune your Position:

■The **ear** lines up over your **shoulder joint**. ■The **shoulder joint** lines up over your **hip joint**. ■**Waistband** lays flat, it does not tilt backward or forward

■For all seated exercises, **your waistband should not tilt backward at all**. ■If it does, **simply raise your hips** up on a firm pillow or mat until you are able to stack up properly. ■The feet stay on the floor. ■ This will allow your pelvis to stack up, putting you in your strongest position.

KEY POSITION: Kneeling

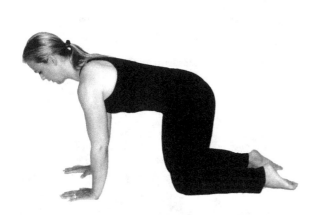

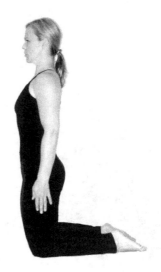

Kneeling Tabletop

■Kneel on your mat, stacking your hips directly over your knees and your shoulders directly over your wrists. ■Flatten your back as much as you can so that you look like a solid tabletop.

Kneeling Upright

■From **Kneeling tabletop,** walk your hands toward your knees and roll the spine upward until you are upright. ■**Stack & Lengthen:** reach your spine toward both the ground and the sky. This will spread out the work of supporting your body.

Anchor Points for Kneeling Positions

a

Kneeling Tabletop

■ **Baseline;** scoop in from hipbone to hipbone.

■ **Ribcage;** knit the ribs inward, as if you were wearing a corset.

■ **Hands, Feet & Shins:** lengthening the arms and legs, gently press the contact points — hands, feet and shins — into your mat. Ever so slightly, push the shin a tiny bit into your mat, as if you wanted to fully extend your leg.

Kneeling Upright

■Baseline ■Ribcage ■Feet & Shins *and...*

■**Seat;** squeeze your bottom.

■**Armpits:** gently draw them toward your hips.

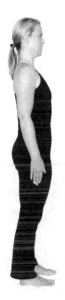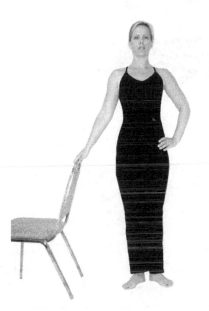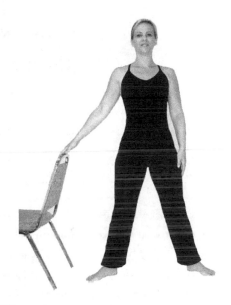

Standing

■**Lengthen** toward both the ground and the sky; this will stabilize the bottom of the stretch, as well as spread the work along the length of your body. ■Keep your anchor points engaged as you lengthen.

Anchor Points
Standing Positions

■ **Baseline;** scoop in from hipbone to hipbone.

■ **Ribcage;** knit the ribs inward, as if you were wearing a corset.

■ **Seat;** squeeze your bottom.

■ **Armpits:** gently draw them toward your hips.

■ **Soles of your feet;** press these into the floor.

Pilates V

This position is borrowed from 1st position in ballet training. ■Stand upright with your heels touching, toes apart. ■Squeeze your seat to help you keep the heels together and create a natural girdle around your hips. ■Draw in at the **Baseline**; lengthen your spine.

Wide Pilates V

■From **Pilates V**, step to the side so that your feet are slightly wider than your shoulders. Maintain your seat squeeze as you lengthen the spine.

KEY POSITION: Prone

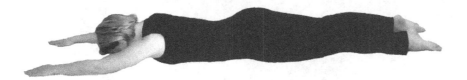

■Lay face down, with your forehead resting on the backs of your hands. Draw your belly button in.

Anchor Points **for Prone Positions**

a

- **Baseline;** scoop in from hipbone to hipbone.
- **Legs;** gently press them into your mat.
- **Armpits;** gently draw them toward your hips. Another way of thinking of this is to draw your shoulders away from your ears *without creating tension near the neck.*

Checkpoint

- **Do not squeeze your Seat in this position.**   Whenever you're considering arching the back even the tiniest bit, do not squeeze your seat, as it may cause undue tension in the low back.

THE ABC'S IN REVIEW

Anchor Points = The Key to Stability

Begin at the beginning: check your Anchor Points first.

- Your body works most efficiently when it has **strong anchors** for each movement, so work toward activating these in every position and every movement. Over time, they'll become second nature. When in doubt, remember: **one body part moves, the rest of the body stays still.**

- If you're already anchoring and you're unable to stay still, **make your range of movement smaller.**

- **Good News:** when you activate your anchor points, you get a two-part benefit. The moving part of your body get more focused work, <u>and</u> your anchor point gets stronger as well.

- **75% Effort** is the perfect amount when you're activating your Anchor Points. In other words, you don't need to squeeze every muscle to its maximum ability. In fact, that will cause new, unnecessary aches and pains.

Body Geometry = Your Best Position

It's not you. Sometimes, the most efficient position *isn't* obvious. Each movement and position will feel simpler and will get more work done when you're using the correct Body Geometry.

■Simply come back to the **Five Basic Shapes and Concepts** that we looked at in this chapter: **Box, Triangle, Level Shoulders, Stack**, and **Lengthen**. ■Your goal is to able to maintain these positions while you're moving. I'll let you know which ones are most important in each exercise. ■Look for tips on how to maintain your best position in the Body Geometry sections throughout this book.

Comfort Options = Fine Tuning Choices

I want you to be comfortable in every position and movement, whether you're exercising or not. If something isn't working for you, it's time to **evaluate and adjust.**

■Choose your key position based on whether it is comfortable for you. ■Choose the size of your movement — your range of motion — based on whether it is comfortable for you. ■Advance to the next position or the next bigger movement size is only when you feel no pain or discomfort, **and** you're able to maintain your anchor points. ■Look for and use the Comfort Options throughout this book.

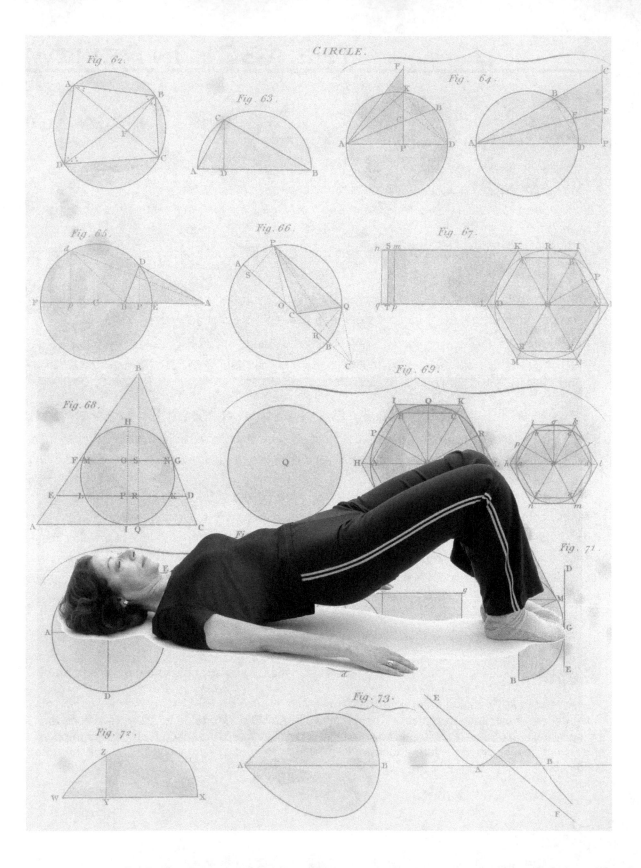

Fig. 62.

Fig. 63.

Fig. 64.

Fig. 65.

Fig. 66.

Fig. 67.

Fig. 68.

Fig. 69.

Fig. 71.

Fig. 72.

Fig. 73.

BUILDING BLOCKS

The movements in this lesson are the building blocks for body awareness and comfort. They are simple enough to be performed by virtually everyone, yet so effective that you will continue to see improvements in your strength, flexibility and range of motion every time you perform them. Amazing!

Do your body a tremendous favor. Commit to a movement lesson of some kind **every day**. Just 15 minutes of focused movement patterns each day will ensure that you maintain and improve a comfortable body that can do what you want it to do.

Need more incentive than that? Experts have found that movement and the breath involved with moving your body are both strong mood elevators. **Your mood will lift in every 15-minute session** and seeing the improvements in your body mechanics will keep that lift going.

LESSON 1: SPINE WARM UP

The Spine Warm Up lesson teaches you how to free up the vertebrae while gently stretching your muscles. You'll use your deep abdominals to move through each position, increasing your strength and flexibility with every movement.

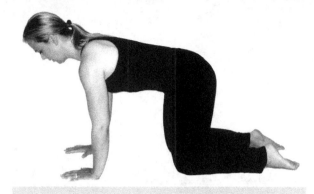

Do All 3 Exercises

- **Pregnant Cat**
- **Cat/Cow**
- **Dogtail**

Begin in Kneeling Tabletop

24

Body Geometry
Tip: How to Breathe

■Blow a Kiss: exhale through gently pursed lips, emptying your lungs completely. When your body craves the next breath, inhale though your nose. ■Synch up your exhale and inhale to match the timing of your movements. Each breath and each movement take the same amount of time.

■Don't worry if this is more difficult than it sounds; take your time.

Anchor Points
for this Lesson

- **Baseline;** scoop in from hipbone to hipbone.
- **Ribcage;** draw the ribs inward, as if you were wearing a corset.
- **Hands, Feet & Shins:** lengthening the arms and legs, gently press the contact points — hands, feet and shins — into your mat. Ever so slightly, push the shin a tiny bit into your mat, as if you wanted to fully extend your leg.

A	B	C
Pregnant Cat	**Cat/Cow**	**Dogtail**

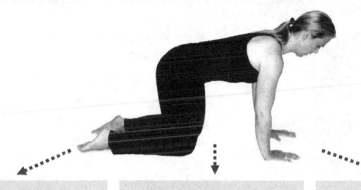

**Relax belly
like a pregnant cat**

Scoop up the Kittens!

Arch Up like a Cat

**Reverse to
Cow position**

**Side Bend
Head and Tail**

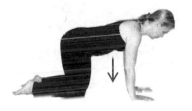 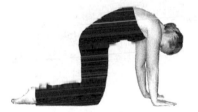 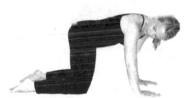

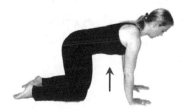 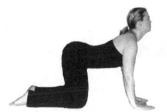

PREGNANT CAT

Pregnant Cat is the great light bulb moment for many people. No matter where you're starting from today, **everyone can access their deep core muscles to 'scoop up the kittens'.**

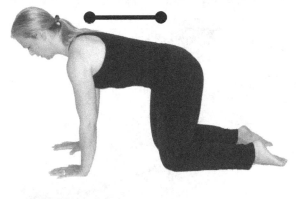

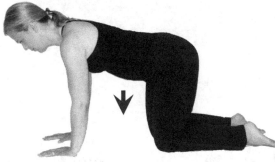

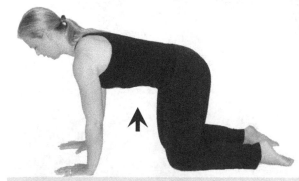

Begin in **Kneeling Tabletop position**

While keeping your back flat, let your belly hang down. The idea is to look like a pregnant cat with a belly full of kittens. ■Without moving your back, scoop up the belly full of kittens. **Draw your stomach up as much as you can.** I know you can move it, even if it's just a little bit. Here's the good news – **you just used your deep abdominal muscles!**

Inhale while you're letting your belly hang. ■How does your low back feel — ache-y, tense? Or does it not feel like much at all?

Exhale as you **scoop up the kittens**. Exhaling gives your body a natural cue to release tension, so take care to <u>not</u> hold your breath. ■**Notice:** how your back feels now. We're shooting for 'relaxed,' or 'less stressed.'

While keeping the kittens scooped up, try inhaling and exhaling. You can breathe while still engaging your abdominal muscles. As you do this more and more, **your lungs and ribcage will expand. sideways**, rather than your belly expanding out.

Body Geometry Tip: Scoop Up the Kittens

Make the phrase **Scoop up the Kittens** a constant in your life --- whenever you step in or out of your car, whenever you lift a child or a sack of groceries, whenever you swing a golf club, **Scoop Up the Kittens.**

CAT/COW

Cat/Cow encourages each tiny bone your spine, to move independently, like the links in a bicycle chain. When the chain moves smoothly, the body feels effortless.

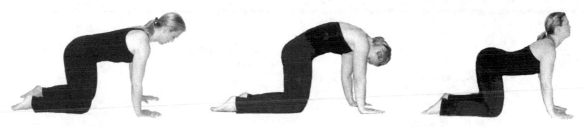

Begin in **Kneeling Tabletop position**

Exhaling, arch your spine up so that you look like a hissing cat. ■Try to move each vertebra individually. Feel your spine s-t-r-e-t-c-h. Let your head hang down comfortably. ■Gently and slowly, rotate your head as if you were saying 'no.' **This creates natural traction of the bones of your neck, opening up space for your discs, which are your body's natural shock absorbers.**

Inhaling, reverse the arch, so that your head and tailbone are higher than your stomach. ■Stretch the belly in this position, while still scooping up the kittens. ■**Create anchors at your armpits so that your shoulders drape down low.** This allows your neck feels loose ■Choose a spot to gaze at that feels comfortable for your neck. **Notice** where that 'easy gaze' is located. **In the following weeks, you may notice that your range of motion increases.** ■Repeat this movement series 5-10x.

 ## Comfort Option: Relief for Sensitive Wrists

■**Try turning your fingertips out <u>slightly</u>** while pressing into your entire palm. This will help evenly distribute your body weight.

■Over time, the natural padding on our hands and feet can thin out leaving us feeling pressure in new and surprising places. **Try rolling up the edge of your mat** or put a thin pillow under the heels of your hands to offer more padding.

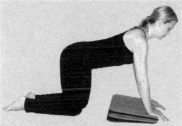

■**Changing your hand position to a fist** can also do the trick. **Be sure to turn your elbow folds forward** when choosing this option. This creates a stacked joint that has more strength to support your weight. Always use padding in this position, as your knuckles have very little natural padding.

DOGTAIL

Dogtail encourages the spine to move in a side bending pattern. When was the last time you moved like this? A healthy spine has the ability to flex to the side, but if you don't move this way, you can lose this ability.

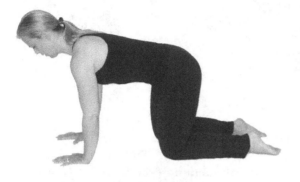

Begin in **Kneeling Tabletop position.** ■Inhale to prepare for the movement.

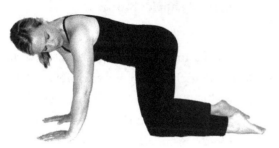

Twist sideways a bit to the right, as you exhale. Bring your head and your tail a little closer together, like a dog looking for his tail. ■Inhale to return to your start position. ■Exhale to look for your tail on the left. ■Notice whether the movement is easier to one side or the other. This may balance out over time; there is no need to force the movements to be identical.

Repeat this movement series 3-5x.

CHILD'S POSE

Child's Pose releases tension in your low back. It gently stretches muscles that may be working a bit too much to support this area of your body. Use it anytime you want to encourage this area to relax.

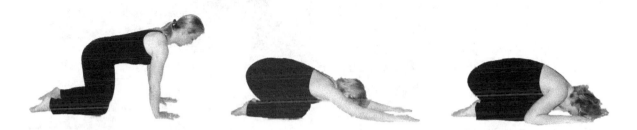

Begin in **Kneeling Tabletop position**

Exhale as you drop your hips back toward your heels. ■Release the weight of your body onto your head and forearms. ■Draw your armpits toward your hips. This increases the stretch along your sides, while taking tension away from your neck. ■Allow your spine and back to gently stretch. ■ Breathe easily in this position for 30 seconds to 5 minutes.

Comfort Options

C

■**If you feel that you need more support**, try using a pillow under your chest to help hold your body weight. This is a good option if your belly or breasts keep you from comfortably resting your weight on your forearms.

■**If your knees do not fold this deeply**, place a small pillow or folded towel at the knee crease, so that you're sitting on it.

■**If your shoulder, neck or upper back feel uncomfortable,** try drawing your elbows back a bit, toward your hips.

■It is ok to open your knees wider, to make more space for your fold-over position.

LESSON 2: PELVIS WARM-UP

In this lesson, we'll begin working on your **Body Geometry** awareness. In the ABC's chapter, you learned that **Balance a Teacup** or 'Neutral Pelvis position' means lining up your pubic bone and hip bones on the same plane. This allows your muscles to work in the most efficient manner. In **Pelvic Tilt** and **Pelvic Clock** we'll work with the interplay of muscles surrounding your pelvis. The awareness that you gain from practicing these movements will give you **control over your body comfort throughout your daily life.**

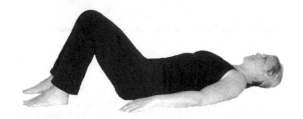

Begin in
Supine/Knees Bent Position 20

Do all 3 of these Exercises

- Pelvic Tilt & Pelvic Clock
- Bridge
- Spine Stretch Forward

Body Geometry
Tip: Scoop Up the Kittens in All Positions

Learning to engage your deep abdominal muscles is often easiest in a Tabletop position with the cue to **Scoop up Kittens**. You can do this any position though! Simply draw in at the bread basket to create an anchor point. This will also support the opposite side of your body: the low back.

Anchor Points
for this Lesson

- **Baseline;** scoop in from hipbone to hipbone.
- **Seat:** squeeze your bottom.
- **Soles of your feet;** press these into the floor.

PERFORM ALL 3 MOVEMENTS

A	B	C
Pelvic Tilt & Clock	Bridge	Spine Stretch Forward

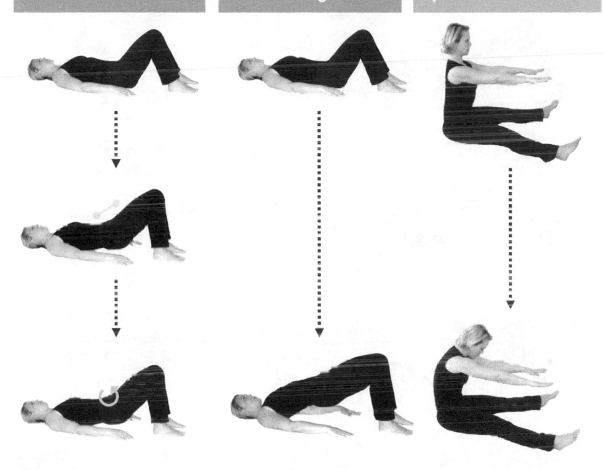

PELVIC TILT

Pelvic Tilt releases the muscles in your low-back. You'll also begin to notice how you hold and move your pelvis in daily life. The position and movement of your pelvis governs the comfort of your low-back.

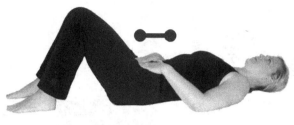

Begin in **Supine/Knees Bent Position**

Place the heels of your hands on hip bones, with your fingertips pointed toward your public bone. Inhale to prepare for the movement.

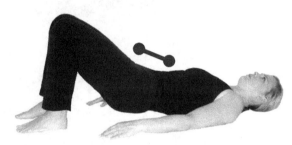

Exhale as you draw your belly button toward the floor. ■Think: **scoop up the kittens**. Your fingertips will now sit higher than your thumbs. ■Notice in the photo: my belly button is now closer to the floor and my hips are tilted upward.

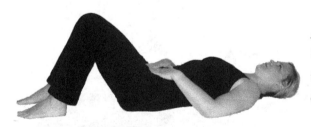

Allow your pelvis to return to its normal position. ■It's ok to release your active scoop here. Over time, try maintaining the scoop throughout each exercise.

Comfort Option: Honor your Lumbar Curve

When laying down, it's ok to have a space between your low back and the floor. This is your natural **lumbar, or low-back curve**. The curves of the spine provide shock absorption and transfer energy where it's needed when we walk and move. It's best to exercise and move with them intact. ■Some people are able to flatten their low back entirely against the floor while performing Pelvic Tilt, and some people cannot. No worries, simply move in that direction, and you'll be doing fine. **There is no need to flatten your back entirely in any exercise.**

PELVIC CLOCK

Pelvic Clock enhances your ability to move the pelvis in many directions. As you increase your range of motion, you'll find that walking and moving in daily life become more comfortable.

Make your movements tiny in this exercise, increasing them a little bit over time.

Begin in **Supine/Knees Bent Position,** with your hands in a triangle.

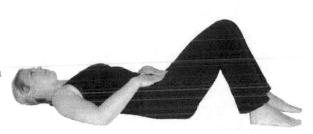

Sink your right hipbone closer to the floor. ■Your right hand will now sit a little lower than your left hand. Think: **scoop up the kittens**.

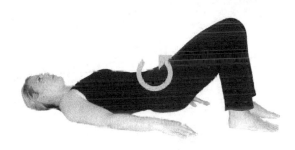

Level out your hips as you draw your belly button toward the floor, as in **Pelvic Tilt.** ■Your fingertips will now sit higher than your thumbs.

■Sink your left hipbone a little closer to the floor. Your left hand will now sit lower than your right hand. ■Return to your start position.

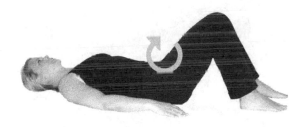

Repeat this movement 3x, then reverse the direction of your **pelvic clock.**

 ## Body Geometry Tip: What about those Tight Spots?

■**Notice** where you have tight spots; where your body might not want to move.
■**Notice** where moving in one direction is easier or more difficult.

This will ease up as your abdominals become stronger. **Give yourself credit for all the little changes you are creating in your body**. Each of these changes will make movement in your daily life more comfortable.

BRIDGE

Bridge is the first exercise that asks you to move an anchor point. You'll scoop up the kittens, and then float them up as you lift your hips. As you master this movement, you'll notice that your legs, hips and abdominals are getting stronger.

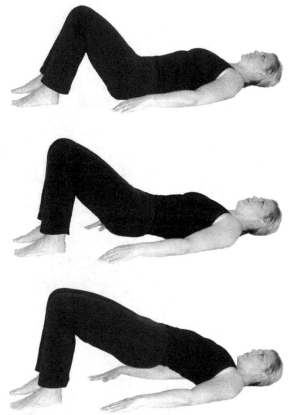

Begin in Supine/Knees Bent Position, with your feet parallel and toes straight forward. Inhale as you lengthen your spine as long as possible. Push your feet into your mat and scoop up the kittens

■Exhale during the movement: tilt your pelvis as in **Pelvic Tilt** and continue until you have lifted your tailbone off the floor. Pause here as you inhale. ■Exhale as you lower back to a neutral spine position.

■Try again, this time peeling one vertebra at a time off the floor until your spine and thighs are in one long line. There is no need to arch, as this may compress your discs. Pause here and inhale. ■Exhale as you lower each vertebra down to your mat. Try to drop each one onto the mat individually. Repeat 5x.

Body Geometry Tip: Be Aware of your Foot Position

■**Notice** whether you **unconsciously lift your toes or heels**, or whether you roll your feet. ■Can you evenly distribute your weight across your feet? ■**Notice** how the movement of your spine now feels.

■**Notice** whether your **knees splay out or tilt in** during the movement. ■Can you keep your knees lined up with your sitting bones? ■Notice how bridging now feels.

EARN BONUS POINTS

Body Geometry Boost: The Power of the Kegal

A 'kegal' is the action where you contract the muscles that would stop or allow the flow of urine. I coach my clients to earn a bonus point by adding a kegal when they 'exhale to move' in an exercise. ■**The best position for Kegals:** moving from a bent hip & knee position to a straight leg.

Kegal exercises lift the pelvic floor, which activates your deep abdominal muscles, and we all need more of that! These muscles support your pelvic organs. Exercising them helps prevent leaking urine when you sneeze or cough, increases sexual enjoyment, can make giving birth easier, and helps to create a sleek lower abdomen.

Kegal & Inner Thigh Booster

■ During Bridge **try squeezing a small pillow or ball between your knees**. For some people, this action helps activate the correct muscles. You may find that you can move further when you include that ball!

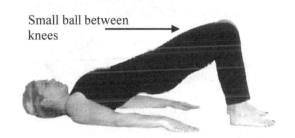

Small ball between knees

Body Geometry Boost: Bridging 3-ways

Bridge 3 Ways: varying the position of your feet in Bridge taxes your muscles from different directions. That's useful in real life when you step on an unstable surface like mud, ice or gravel. You'll be better able to stop yourself from slipping and falling. You've already tried bridge with **Feet Parallel**, ■now try it with your feet turned out like a **duck**. This will engage your seat and the muscles on the outside of your legs. ■Next, try it with your feet turned in like a **pigeon**. This will engage your inner thighs more. Be careful to still keep your knees lined up with your hips.

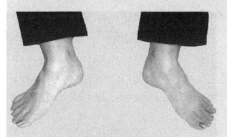

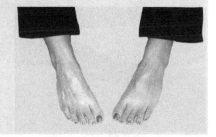

SPINE STRETCH FORWARD

Spine Stretch Forward creates pockets of space for the discs that sit between each of your vertebrae. Discs are part of your body's natural shock absorption system. They act like little puffed up sponges that protect the bones of your spine. Creating space between them allows for maximum shock absorption and maximum comfort in your daily life.

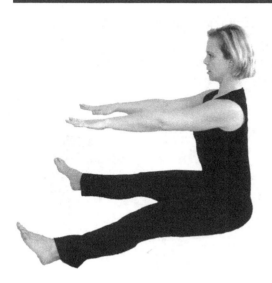

Begin in **Sitting Upright/Legs Extended** position. Open your legs to a wide V. Inhale, as you squeeze your seat and try to grow an inch taller. Squeezing your seat creates an important Anchor Point in all seated exercises.

■Exhale as you float your arms straight in front of you. Anchor your armpits low. ■Envision that you have placed your hands on a large ball in front of you.

■Inhale. Exhale as you scoop in the kittens and round your spine. ■Envision that you are using your **abdominal muscles** to press the ball down. Inhale to sit tall again. ■Repeat 5x.

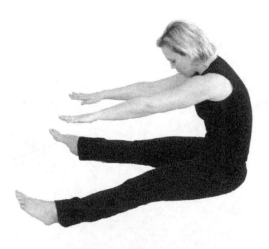

a   Anchor Points for this Lesson

- **Baseline;** scoop in from hipbone to hipbone.
- **Seat;** squeeze your bottom.
- **Soles of your feet;** press these into the floor.

As we move to upright, the torso must anchor itself more, without the aid of the mat. So, we add:

- **Ribcage;** knit the ribs inward, as if you were wearing a corset.

■**For all Seated Exercises** your hip bones need to float directly over your sitting bones. The easy way to check for this: **your waist band should not be tipping backward,** as seen in the photo to the right.

When you cannot sit upright in this position, the backs of your legs are likely a bit tight.

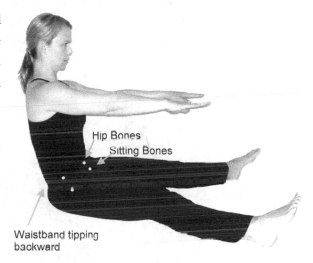

Hip Bones

Sitting Bones

Waistband tipping backward

Comfort Option:
Don't Struggle to Sit Tall

■**Try sitting up on a mat** that lifts your hips 2-3 inches higher. This will position your hips higher than your legs, so that the tight leg muscles do not pull your pelvis out of alignment.

■**Nothing available to sit up on?** Bend your knees and put your feet flat on your mat. Ageless Pilates exercises will help you stretch your body where it has become tight. With practice, **you will gain flexibility.**

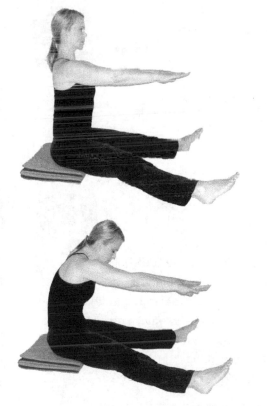

LESSON 3: SHOULDER WARM-UP

The Shoulder Warm-up lesson often causes spontaneous relief from neck and upper back tension. This is Body Geometry at its best. As your body learns to position your shoulder blades well, and to begin arm movement from this area, your upper body movement will feel effortless.

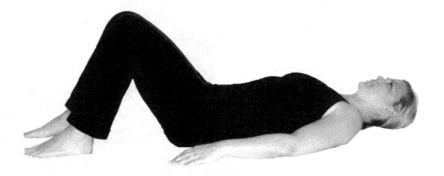

Try All 3 Exercises, Choose 1 that feels Best

Begin in Supine/Knees Bent Position 20

- Puppet Arms
- Ribcage Arms
- Arm Circles

Body Geometry
Tip: Melt Away Neck

Many people carry their tension in their neck and shoulders. ■Whenever you feel tension creeping into this area, **melt your armpits toward your hips**, and slowly turn your head from side to side. ■ This will help bring you back to your most comfortable body geometry.

 Anchor Points for this Lesson

- **Baseline;** scoop in from hipbone to hipbone.
- **Seat:** squeeze your bottom.
- **Soles of your feet;** press these into the floor.

CHOOSE YOUR LEVEL OF COMFORT

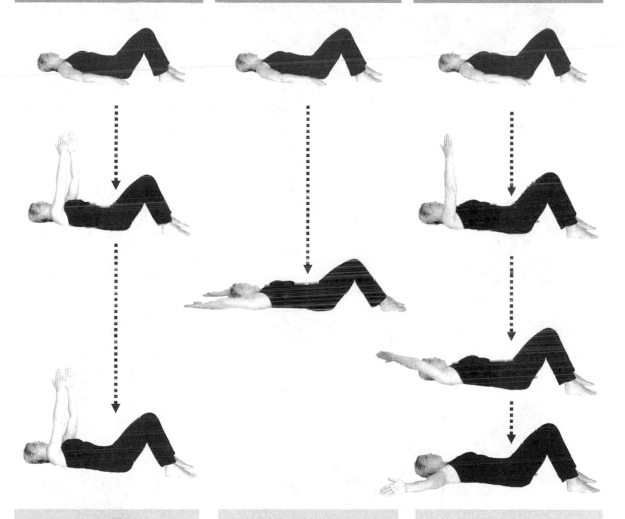

A	B	C
Puppet Arms	**Ribcage Arms**	**Arm Circles**

Lift the shoulder blades off the mat

Lower them back onto the mat

With shoulders away from the ears, float the arms up & back

With shoulders away from the ears, draw circles with the arms

PUPPET ARMS

Puppet Arms awakens your shoulder blade awareness. You'll notice neck tension melting away as you learn to drop your shoulder blades back onto the mat.

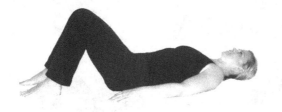

Begin this exercise in Supine/Knees Bent Position. Inhale as you lengthen your spine as long as possible.

■Exhale as you draw your armpits toward your hips. This movement is small and subtle. It's ok if there is no actual movement, as long you are trying to feel your armpits sinking low. ■Inhale, keeping your armpits low.

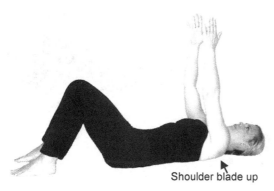
Shoulder blade up

■Exhale as you float your arms up until your fingertips point toward the sky. Are you armpits still low? Inhale again. ■Exhale as you peel your shoulder blades off the mat. Feel the space between your shoulder blades become wide. ■ Inhale as you lower your shoulder blades back down.

Repeat 5x

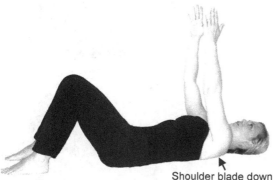
Shoulder blade down

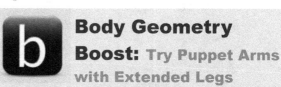
Body Geometry Boost: Try Puppet Arms with Extended Legs

■Flatten both out while keeping your pelvis in neutral. ■Can you keep your pelvis steady while moving your arms?

■The torso must remain 'quiet' or still during this exercise. **This is your test to determine whether it's time to progress to the straight-leg variation.**

RIBCAGE ARMS & ARM CIRCLES

Ribcage Arms adds a bit of chest stretch to the movement pattern that you learned with Puppet Arms. You'll feel new muscles awakening as you control the urge to arch your back when your arms are moving. When this movement pattern carries into your daily life, neck tension will continue to melt away.

Begin this exercise in Supine/Knees Bent Position with your arms long and loose beside you. Inhale as you lengthen your spine as long as possible

■Exhale as you float your arms up and back in the direction of your ears. Move slowly, keeping your armpits low and your shoulder blades on your mat. ■If your shoulder begins to pull up toward your ear, you've gone too far for today. ■Inhale, as you bring your arms back to your start position.

Repeat this movement 5x.

■Note when your arm movement starts to cause your pelvis to shift, tipping your imaginary teacup. Try scooping in a little deeper to **counteract any tipping**. As you continue to practice this movement, your range of motion will increase.

Now try this movement one arm at a time. ■**Notice** whether you can move one arm further than the other. Your range of motion will likely increase over time.

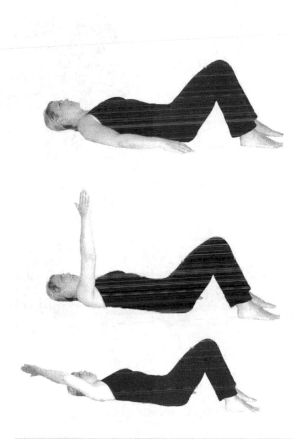

b

Body Geometry
Boost: Try Arm Circles

Continue the movement by sliding your extended arms along the mat, back to your hips, similar to making a snow angle. Feel your shoulder blades slide further down your back.

LESSON 4: LEG & HIP WARM-UP

The Leg and Hip warm-up lesson encourages you to maintain a neutral pelvis position while moving your legs. Many people find that this new awareness translates to relief from low back pain in their daily life.

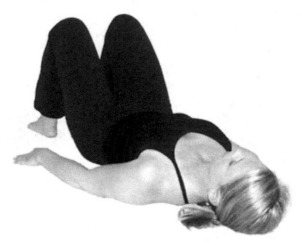

Try All 4 Exercises, Choose 2 that feel Best	**Begin in Supine/Knees Bent Position** 20

- Leg Slides
- Knee Drops
- Knee Drop & Drag
- Low Back Release

 Anchor Points for this Lesson

- **Baseline;** scoop in from hipbone to hipbone.
- **Seat:** squeeze your bottom.
- **Soles of your feet;** press these into the floor.

A	B	C
Leg Slides	**Knee Drops**	**Knee Drop & Drag**

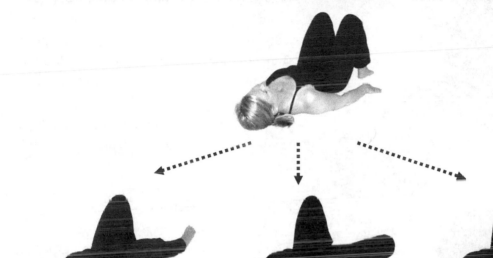

Extend one leg from Bent to flat

Drop one knee sideways

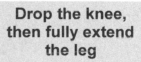

Drop the knee, then fully extend the leg

Body Geometry Tip:

Quiet your Torso — keep it still — throughout these movements

If this should become difficult:
- Check your **Anchor Points**;
- Make your **Range of Movement** smaller until you are able to stabilize your torso.

LEG SLIDES

This mind-body coordination movement challenges your ability to keep your pelvis steady, a key piece of Body Geometry. Learning new movement patterns like this builds neural pathways in the brain, which helps to keep your mind agile.

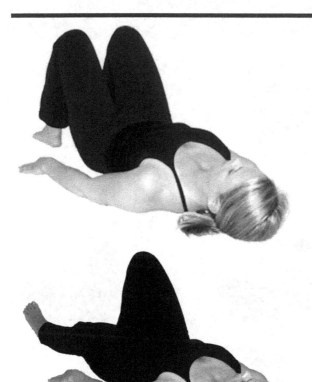

Begin this exercise in **Supine/Knees Bent Position**. Inhale as you lengthen your spine. ■Scoop up the kittens and exhale as you **push your right foot as if it were moving through sand**, until your leg is fully extended. Inhale to prepare for the next movement. ■Exhale as you drag your right foot through the sand, back to your starting position. ■Repeat with the left leg.

Repeat 5-10x on each leg.

■**Notice** whether this movement is easier or more difficult with one leg than the other. Differences between the two legs will lessen as you continue to practice this movement.

Body Geometry Boost: Try these Variations

■Test your **neutral pelvis position** by trying this exercise with your hands forming a triangle on your lower abdomen. Your imaginary teacup should sit level on the triangle

■When this movement begins to seem easy, try moving both legs at the same time. Mentally check in: are you able to balance the imaginary teacup throughout the movement?

KNEE DROPS

It's fun to try different movement patterns and to notice where your body is more or less coordinated. Sometimes, introducing a new pattern also means extending your comfort range.

Begin this exercise in **Supine/Knees Bent Position**. Inhale as you lengthen your spine. ■ Scoop up the kittens and exhale as you **lower your right knee to the side, toward the floor**. The bottom of your foot will come off of the floor in this position. ■Exhale as you draw the knee back to your start position. ■Repeat the movement with your left leg.

Repeat 5-10x on each leg.

■**Notice** whether you can you lower your leg all the way to the floor, while staying in neutral pelvis position. No worries — the range of motion in your hip will increase over time. Inhale to prepare for the next movement.

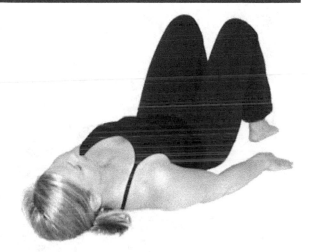

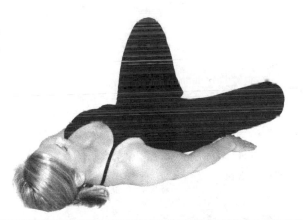

Body Geometry Tip:
Direct your Energy Toward your Movement
■Keep your feet relaxed during these exercises; there is no need to point or flex either foot. ■Adding effort where it isn't needed can create a habit of holding extra tension in the body. This drains you of energy and can create more wear on your body than is necessary.

KNEE DROP & DRAG

Combining several movements adds more challenge for the brain. Mastering new patterns like this translates to more graceful movement in your daily life.

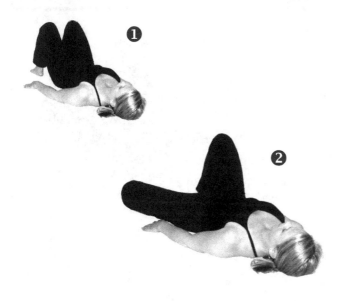

Begin this exercise in **Supine/Knees Bent Position**. Inhale as you lengthen your spine. ■Scoop up the kittens and exhale as you drop your right knee to the side, toward the floor. Inhale to prepare for the movement. ■Exhale as you push your outside ankle through sand, extending your leg forward. Keep your leg turned out until it is fully extended.

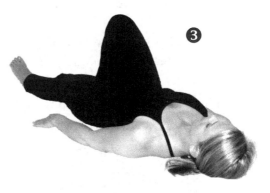

■**Inhale** as you rotate your thigh so that your knee points skyward. ■**Exhale** as you drag your foot back to your start position. Repeat with your left leg.

Repeat 5-10x on each leg.

■**Notice** whether one leg moves more easily than the other. Many people feel a difference from one side to the other; this will balance out as you continue to practice.

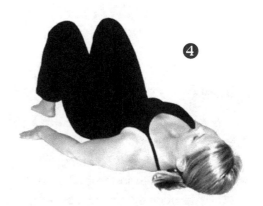

LOW BACK RELEASE

This simple position gently rotates and releases the spine.

Begin this exercise in Supine/**Knees Bent Position**. Inhale as you lengthen your spine. ■Scoop up the kittens and exhale as you lower both knees toward the right, allowing your pelvis to move freely. It's ok if your shoulders shift, this one isn't an exact science. ■Slowly inhale and exhale several times in this position. ■Inhale as you draw the knees back to your start position. ■Repeat on your left side.

■**Notice** whether you are able to move more comfortably to one side than the other. This is common; your range of motion will change over time.

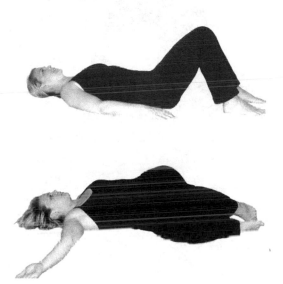

Comfort Options

■Would you feel more comfortable with a pillow to bolster up your knees? If so, use one. Never force your body into an uncomfortable position, as this is one of the habits that leads to compensation patterns.

■Whatever you practice while doing Pilates becomes a habit in your everyday life. Avoid gripping your muscles to support your body. ■Look for ways to position and move yourself comfortably, while maintaining good Body Geometry.

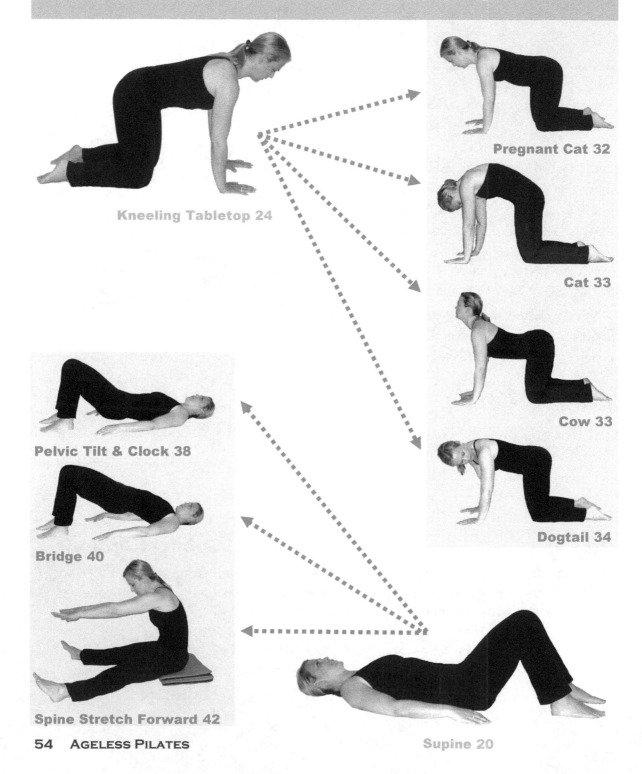

Kneeling Tabletop 24

Pregnant Cat 32

Cat 33

Cow 33

Dogtail 34

Pelvic Tilt & Clock 38

Bridge 40

Spine Stretch Forward 42

Supine 20

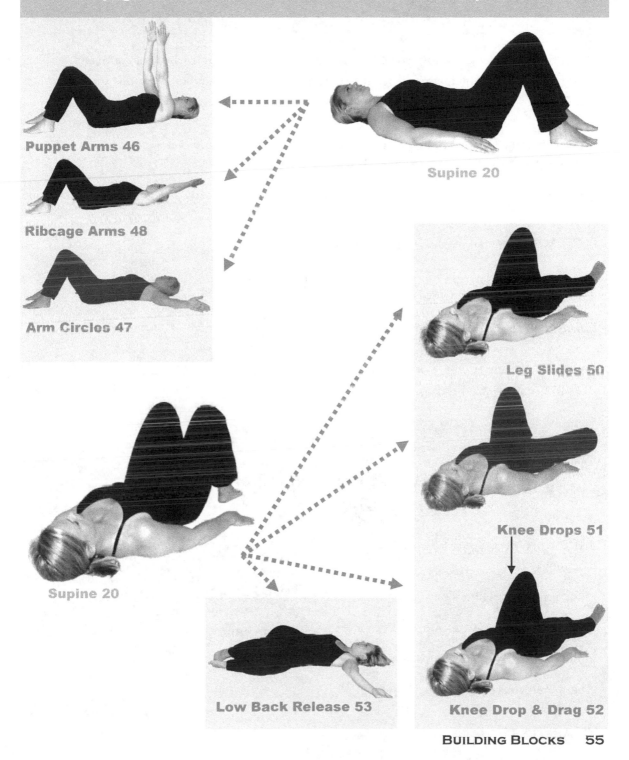

Perform each movement group 5x, then move on to the next group. Use the page numbers to check instructions & anchor points.

Puppet Arms 46

Ribcage Arms 48

Arm Circles 47

Supine 20

Leg Slides 50

Knee Drops 51

Supine 20

Low Back Release 53

Knee Drop & Drag 52

WORKOUT 2: STARFISH

When you've mastered starfish, you'll feel like you've graduated to a new level of coordination. This movement is usually quite a challenge for your motor system to handle, so try this on a day when you feel like you can laugh at yourself.

Begin in **Supine/Knees Bent position**. Scoop up the kittens; slide your right leg out to flat; float your left arm back by your ear. (Opposite arm and leg are extended)

Inhale to prepare for the movement. Exhale as you move **both arms** and **both legs** at the same time:

■Float the right knee up as the left leg extends out to flat;

■Slide the left arm out to the side, as the right arm floats up and back to your ear. ■This is similar to a swimmer's backstroke pattern.

Inhale to prepare, exhale as you switch the arms and legs again.

Repeat 10x

Body Geometry Tips

■The **torso stays quiet** as the arms and legs move.

■Lengthen your spine along your mat.

■Envision pushing water away with your legs and arms; pretend they are moving through something thick and heavy.

■Lengthen your arms and legs during the movement.

Anchor Points for this Lesson

■ **Baseline;** scoop in from hipbone to hipbone.
■ **Ribcage;** knit the ribs inward, as if you were wearing a corset.
■ **Armpits:** envision them melting toward your hips. Do not allow the shoulders to slide up by your ears.

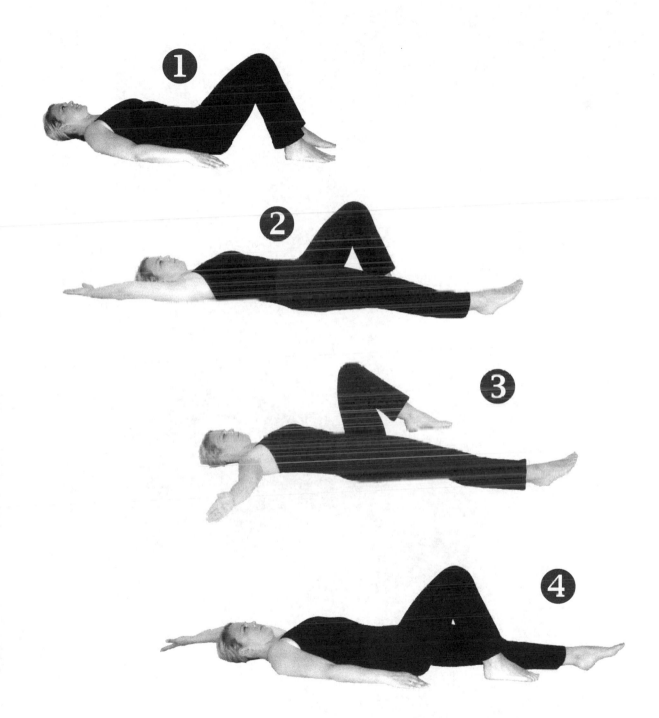

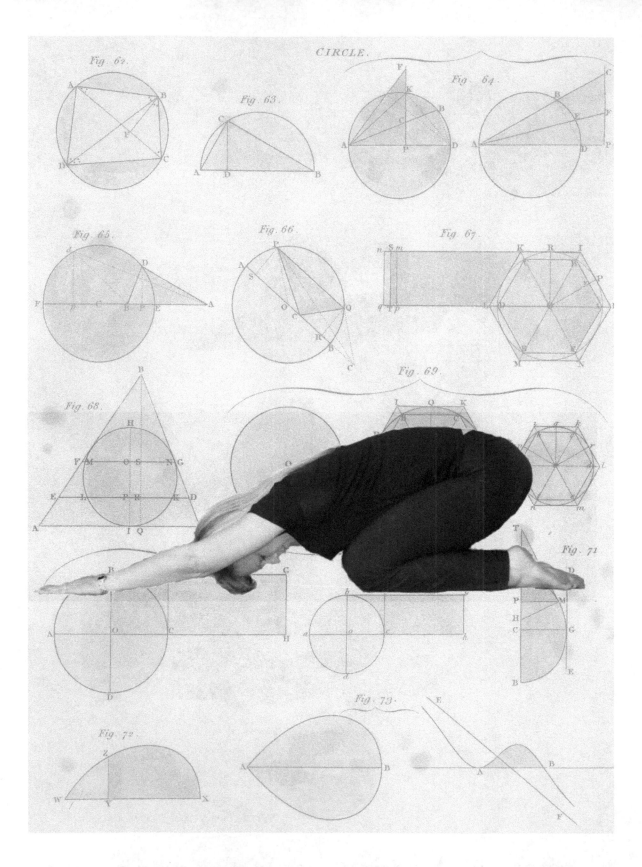

Fig. 62.

Fig. 63.

Fig. 64.

Fig. 65.

Fig. 66.

Fig. 67.

Fig. 68.

Fig. 69.

Fig. 71.

Fig. 72.

Fig. 73.

MATWORK BASICS

This routine is the core of what I personally practice every day. It combines moves from our earlier Lessons with an additional key movement concept: Core Stabilization.

Imagine a child's see-saw. If you put a large adult on one side and a tiny child on the other, you'd need to fiddle around with the center point to make the see-saw work properly. Large movements with your arms and legs require the same focus on the center point of your body, your Core. Once you have your body in its ideal alignment, using Body Geometry, it's a matter of building strength in the core to maintain your position. We call this Core Stabilization.

Do these moves every day, for the rest of your life, and you'll maintain a comfortable range of motion and the ability to move freely. Add other routines from the book as you see fit. Don't be surprised if you become inspired to become more active or to resume a sport or activity that you once enjoyed.

LESSON 5: LEG & HIP MOVES

The Leg and Hip Moves lesson teaches you how to stretch and strengthen your hips and legs, while encouraging your thigh bones to sit properly in your hip socket. In daily life, this makes for loose and easy movement in your hips and a comfortable walking gait.

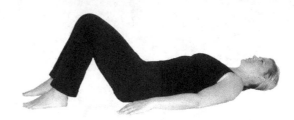

Choose 1 Strength + 1 Stretch move

Begin in Supine/Knees Bent Position 20

- Knee Stirs
- Leg Circles for Strength
- Leg Circles for Stretch
- Hamstring Stretch

Body Geometry Tip:

Anchor Points for this Lesson

Quiet your Torso throughout these movements

If this should become difficult:
- Check your **Anchor Points**;
- Make your **Range of Movement** smaller until you are able to stabilize your torso.

- **Baseline;** scoop in from hipbone to hipbone.
- **Seat:** squeeze your bottom.
- **Soles of your feet;** press these into the floor.

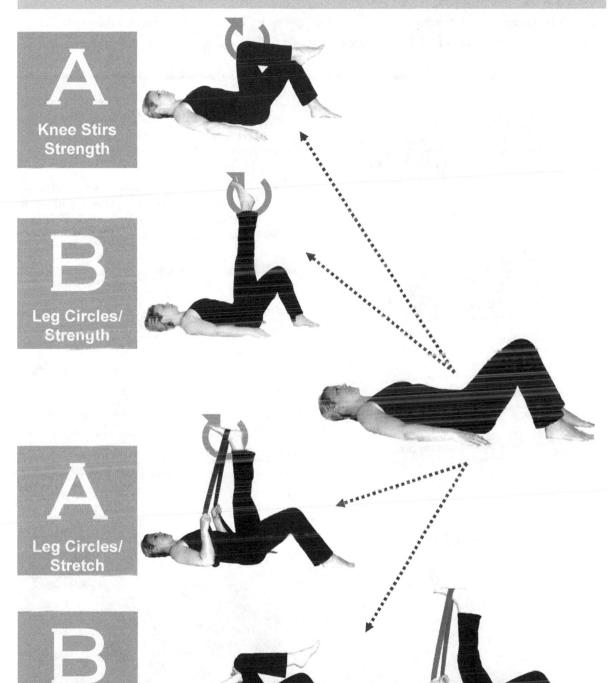

A — Knee Stirs Strength

B — Leg Circles/ Strength

A — Leg Circles/ Stretch

B — Hamstring Stretch

KNEE STIRS

Knee Stirs energize the hip joint by stretching the muscles around the hip and distributing synovial fluid, your body's natural joint lubricant. Well lubricated joints have an easy, juicy feel to them.

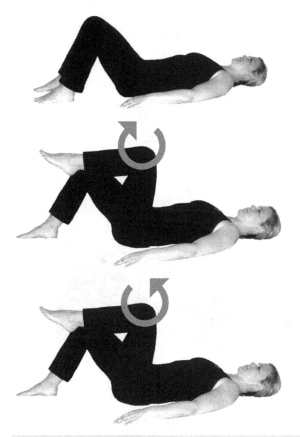

Begin in **Supine/Knees Bent Position.** Inhale to lengthen your spine. Exhale to scoop up the kittens and float your **right knee** toward the sky. Inhale to prepare for the next movement.

■Exhale, drawing a clockwise circle in the air with your knee. Time your movement with your exhale, so that they synch up exactly. ■Repeat 5x clockwise, then 5x counter clockwise.

Repeat with your left leg.

■Is the movement is easier for one of your legs? ■Can you draw bigger circles with one leg? ■Is the movement easier in one direction? ■Many people find differences between the way one leg moves, and the way their other leg moves. As you continue to practice, these differences will lessen.

Comfort Option: Use a Prop

■Try knee stirs with a towel or flex band wrapped around your thigh. Let your leg be a dead weight, and use your arm muscles to move the weight of the leg. ■Can you draw a larger circle this way, while keeping your pelvis in neutral? Doing the movement this way can be very helpful if you tend to carry tension in your hips.

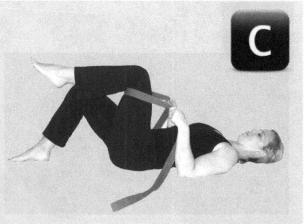

LEG CIRCLES FOR STRETCH

Leg Circles for Stretch ask for a greater range of motion than a knee stir, stretching your muscles a bit more. Performing this movement will help you maintain flexibility and range of motion for your daily life. You may find yourself moving and walking with greater ease.

Begin in **Supine/Knees Bent Position.** Loop a towel, strap or flex band at your right arch. Inhale to lengthen your spine.

■Exhale to scoop up the kittens and **extend your leg toward the sky**, using the band to support the weight of your leg. ■Feel your leg drop into your hip socket. ■Use the Anchor Points at your armpits to weight down your extended leg. Inhale to prepare for the next movement.

■Exhale as you circle your leg, moving clockwise and crossing the body. **Power the movement with your arm muscles.** ■Time your movement with your exhale, so that they synch up exactly. ■Draw 5 circles clockwise, inhaling in-between each circle. Draw 5 circles counter clockwise.

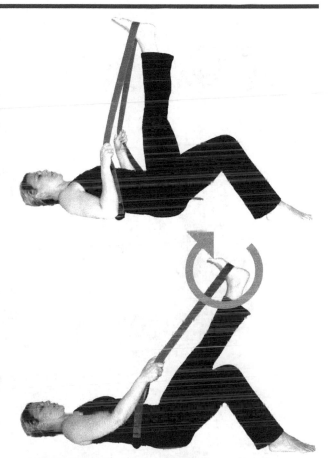

Anchor Points for this Lesson

■Baseline ■Seat
■Sole of your foot *and...*

■ **Armpits & Shoulder Blades;** root them into your mat to anchor the movement of the strap and leg.

Body Geometry Tip

Allow your leg to rotate during the movement: the knee points out to the side when the leg is to the side, the knee points inward when the leg crosses the body.

LEG CIRCLES FOR STRENGTH

Leg Circles for Strength build core, hip and leg strength, all musts for good standing balance.

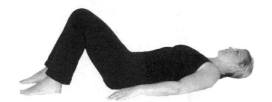

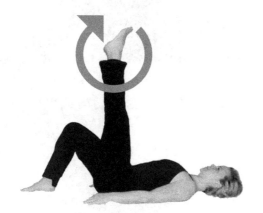

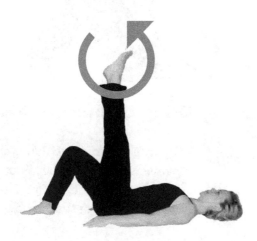

Begin in **Supine/Knees Bent Position.** Inhale to lengthen your spine. ■Exhale to you scoop up the kittens and **float your right leg toward the sky**. Feel your leg drop into your hip socket. Inhale to prepare for the next movement.

■Exhale as you circle your leg, moving clockwise. **Power the movement with your leg muscles.** This will feel very differently than when you used the towel to support the weight of the leg. Make the movement take the same amount of time as it takes you to exhale slowly.

■Time your movement with your exhale, so that they synch up exactly. ■Draw 5 circles clockwise, inhaling in-between each circle. Draw 5 circles counter clockwise.

Repeat with your left leg.

Body Geometry Boost: Try keeping your Anchor Leg Ex-

Your test is whether the torso can stay entirely still. It's ok to make your circles smaller to accomplish this.

HAMSTRING STRETCH

This technique does an amazing job of lengthening the back of your legs without pain. Like all stretching techniques, you do need to perform it on a regular basis to maintain your flexibility.

Measuring your Hamstrings

Begin in Supine/Knees Bent Position. Loop a towel at your right arch. ■Straighten your leg and lift it toward the sky as far as it will comfortably go. ■Make a mental note of where your foot is along the ceiling. Put the towel aside for

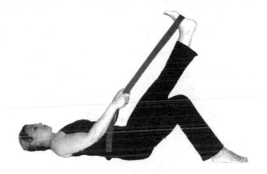

Stretching your Hamstrings:

■Bend your right knee toward your right shoulder, and place both hands against that upper thigh. Inhale to prepare.

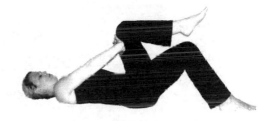

■As you exhale, push your hands against your right thigh and your thigh against your hands. Keep your left foot anchored on the floor. ■Make your exhale take as long as possible; count to ten s-l-o-w-l-y. ■Stop the pushing movement while you inhale. ■Repeat your ten-second exhale again, pushing your hands against your thigh and your thigh against your hands. Inhale to relax.

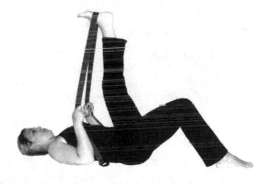

■Measure your hamstring flexibility with the towel again. ■**Notice** whether you can lift your straightened leg higher. ■Repeat on your left leg, . Any differences will balance out greatly as you continue to practice.

C Comfort Option: How often can I do this?

This stretch technique can be repeated on the same leg several times. Once you get to a point where your flexibility isn't improving with repetition, let it go for that day. There is a limit to the amount of change you can create in one day. You'll see even more changes as you continue to practice this regularly.

LESSON 6: BALANCING ABDOMINALS

The Balancing Abdominals lesson is famous for creating fluidity in your spine. You'll ask each of the vertebrae to move independently by tapping into all of the muscle fibers in your abdominals. Some of those fibers have likely been out on vacation. When you've called them all back, you'll be moving like a graceful cat.

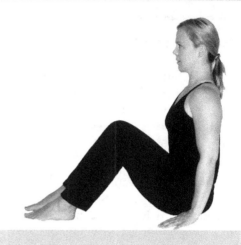

Choose one Rolling move + one Sit-up style move

Begin in Seated/Knees Bent Position 22

- Cradle
- Rocking Cradle
- Rolling Ball

- Roll Up
- Roll Down
- Wall Roll up

Comfort Option:
use a prop

Sometimes, the belly or breasts are in the way; or your knees or hips are not able to bend enough to allow you to hold your thighs. Be creative, **use a prop!** ■ Simply loop a towel or band around your thighs and hold that with your hands.

 ### Anchor Points for this Lesson

- **Baseline;** scoop in from hipbone to hipbone.
- **Seat;** squeeze your bottom.
- **Soles of your feet;** press these into the floor.

As we move to upright, the torso must anchor itself more, without the aid of the mat. So, we add:

- **Ribcage;** knit the ribs inward, as if you were wearing a corset.

A
Cradle

B
Ball

C
Roll Up & Down

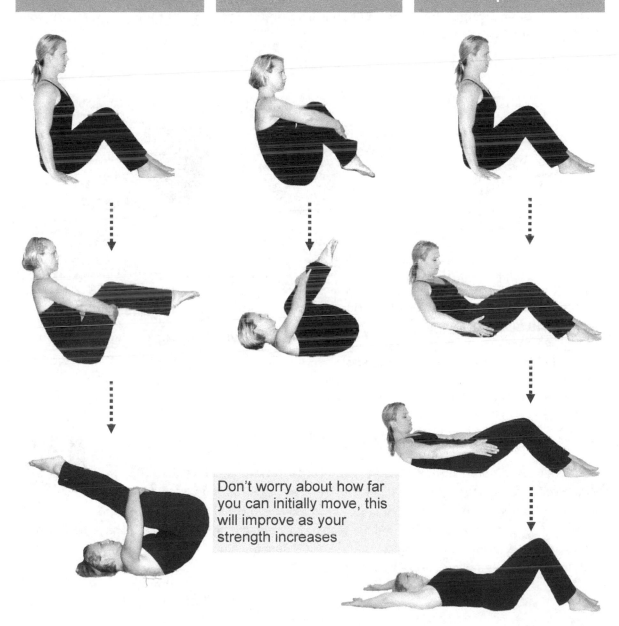

Don't worry about how far you can initially move, this will improve as your strength increases

ROCKING CRADLE

The massaging movement of Rocking Cradle can help to loosen a stiff spine by encouraging each vertebra to move independently. As you rock, you'll feel your deep abdominal muscles working to move through each position. One day, you'll be able to perform this movement in slow-motion.

Begin in **Sitting Upright Position.** Lift your heels and use your hands to hold the back of your thighs up. Inhale, scooping up the kittens.

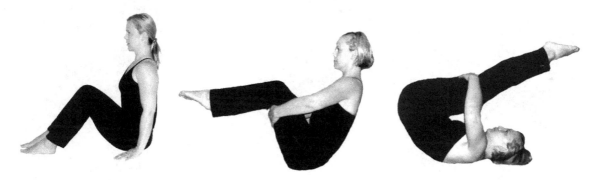

■Exhale as you lift your toes off the floor. Continue scooping up the kittens to keep yourself balanced, like a cradle poised to rock. ■**Notice that your abdominals are working to hold you in this position.**

Simply holding yourself in this **Cradle position** is an exercise in itself. ■Feel how your powerhouse needs to work to hold you in this pose.

■Exhale as you kick your shins up, allowing your body to roll back.   Keep holding onto your thighs! ■Inhale, pull in your scoop a little deeper, and roll back up to your start position.

Repeat 5-10x

Body Geometry Tip: About Discs

Your body has natural shock absorbers called **Discs** between each vertebra. When you have space for them to be plump, like a saturated sponge, your spine feels comfortable. When your vertebrae are too close together or are not moving freely, those sponges are squished tight, leading to an uncomfortable spine. The action of **articulating your spine,** or moving one vertebra at a time frees up the space between each vertebra, helping you keep your discs in good health.

ROLLING LIKE A BALL

Rolling like a Ball requires more abdominal strength than Rocking Cradle — your abdominals must do the work rather than allowing the force of momentum to do the work for you.

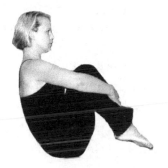 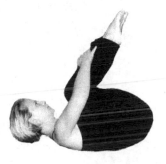 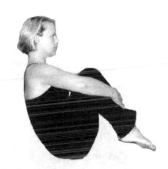

Begin in **Sitting Upright Position** with your heels lifted, and arms wrapped around your thighs.

Inhale, scooping up the kittens. ■Exhale as you push yourself backward with your toes. Scoop in the kittens to assist you in rolling backward. ■Inhale and immediately rock forward to your start position.

■When rolling like a ball becomes easy, try holding a small pillow or rolled up hand towel between your knees.

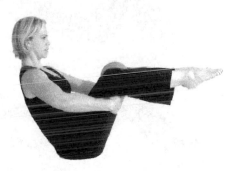

BENT KNEE ROLL-DOWN

The Bent Knee Roll-Down is a powerful abdominal exercise. When you tap into the strength that comes from your anchor points, you may surprise yourself by moving farther than you thought possible. Enjoy your new-found strength, and notice how lovely your back is beginning to feel.

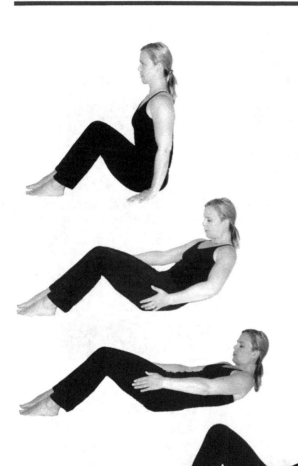

Begin in **Sitting Upright Position** ■Inhale as you scoop up the kittens and lengthen your spine.

■Exhale during the movement. Push your feet into your mat as you round your spine **halfway to the mat.** Keep your spine as long as possible, changing the shape of it from tall to rounded. ■Inhale as you pause in this halfway position.

Exhaling, continue to push your feet into your mat. Scoop up the kittens a little more. ■**Roll up with control** until you reach your start position, sitting tall. ■It's ok to use the strength of your arms to help you climb back up!

As you continue to practice Rolling Down, try increasing the movement all the way down to lying flat on the mat. ■Only come down to the point where you think you can return to your starting position.

Inefficient Movement Alert!

Lifting your feet during roll-ups or roll-downs is considered an **Inefficient Movement** because it incorporates extra muscles — your hip flexors.

■Keep your feet anchored down on your mat to work the abdominal wall. This will flatten your belly.

BENT KNEE ROLL-UP

At first glance, the Bent Knee Roll-Up appears similar to a traditional sit up. When performed Ageless Pilates-style, this movement incorporates many more accessory muscles than a sit-up. Accessory Muscles are the unsung heroes that support your spine in daily life. When they are doing their job, the larger muscles have more energy to perform larger movements.

Begin in **Supine/Knees Bent Position.** Push your feet into the mat and scoop up the kittens.

■Lead with breastbone as you begin to roll up, peeling your shoulder blades off the mat. ■ Grasp your upper thighs as soon as you can reach them. Inhale as you pause **halfway up**.

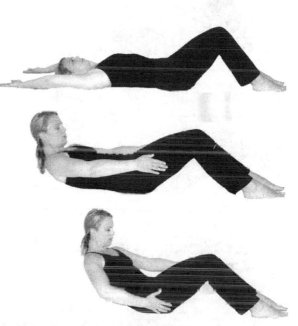

Exhaling, push your feet into the mat as you scoop up the kittens a bit more. ■Roll down with control, printing one vertebrae at a time onto your mat.

■Try increasing the movement until your can sit all the way up.

The Magic of 50/50's

■Each time you practice your Roll-downs, come a little closer to the floor. ■Each time you practice your Roll-ups, come a little closer to upright.

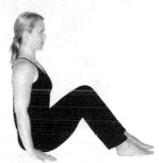

I call these **50/50's**. One day, you'll be rolling all the way down and all the way up. **Remember, little improvements each day will accumulate over time.**

Inefficient Movement Alert!

Using momentum by throwing your body forward is an **Illegal Move**. Momentum doesn't train your abdominals to become stronger. It can tweak your back, which can be discouraging. **Set yourself up for success by being deliberate in your movements.** Give yourself credit for the amount of movement you can muster today, and reach a little bit farther each day.

WALL ROLL-UP

This handy movement trick often helps my clients find the strength to move through a full Roll-Up for the first time. The action of simultaneously pushing your lower body into the floor and the wall gives you a larger anchor point for the movement. You *can* do a full Roll-Up.

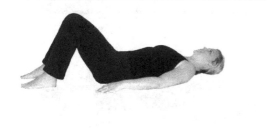

Begin this exercise in Supine/Knees Bent Position. Press your feet flat against a wall, with your thighs at an angle and your toes slightly lower than your knees. ■Inhale as you lengthen your spine and press your hips against your mat.

■Envision your ribcage as a wheel that is about to roll. ■Exhale as you reach for the sky, and roll your ribcage up off the mat. ■Grasp your thighs if you need to; it's ok to climb up your legs. ■Inhale as you pause in your upright position. ■Exhale as you roll back down.

Repeat this movement 5x.

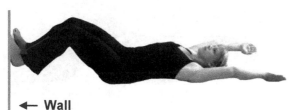

← Wall

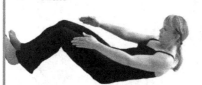

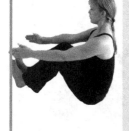

Body Geometry Success Tips

This movement sequence usually requires some fine tuning to get the position perfect for your body. **Here are the 3 things that I'd look at if I were there with you:**

■**Are your thighs at an angle?** If your hips are too close to the wall, this movement becomes more difficult. Try moving your hips a smidge further away from the wall.

■**Are your feet staying against the wall?** If the heels or toes raise, some of your abdominal muscles will take a vacation. Use your leg muscles to push the feet flat against the wall.
■**Can you reach your thighs with your hands?** Try looping a towel behind your thighs, holding the ends in your hands. Use your arms to help you climb up the legs.

This is like walking and chewing gum; there are many things happening at once. No worries if it take a few tries; you can do it!

LESSON 7: SHOULDER PLACEMENT

The Shoulder Placement lesson teaches you how to combat a common tension pattern in our modern culture: **forward-rounded shoulders**. When I see shoulders that are rounded forward or riding high toward the ears, I know exactly where that person's body tension is centered – in their neck and upper back! The two simple exercises in this lesson can draw your shoulders into their optimal alignment, eliminating neck and upper back tension.

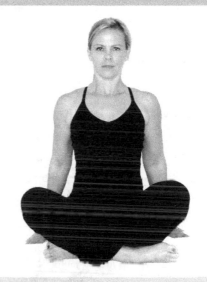

Do Both Exercises

- Dumbwaiter
- Wings

Begin Sitting Upright in a Chair, or Sitting Cross Legged

 Body Geometry Tip: Why we breathe & move this way

Exhaling gives the body the cue to *relax*.

Exhaling during the work phase of an exercise encourages the body to let go of unnecessary tension. This preserves energy, so that you can spend it elsewhere.

 Anchor Points for this Lesson

- **Baseline;** scoop in from hipbone to hipbone.
- **Seat;** squeeze your bottom.
- **Ribcage;** knit the ribs inward, as if you were wearing a corset.

If seated in a chair, add:

- **Soles of your feet;** press these into the floor.

DUMBWAITER

Dumbwaiter is an excellent movement for anyone who feels that their shoulders slump forward even a tiny bit. It trains your body to pull the shoulder blades toward each other, which gives you a dancer's posture: an open chest with relaxed shoulders.

Begin this exercise either sitting tall in a chair or sitting cross legged. ■Glue your elbows to your ribcage and float your hands up as if you were balancing a teacup on your palm. ■Inhale as you scoop up the kittens, squeeze your seat and lengthen your spine.

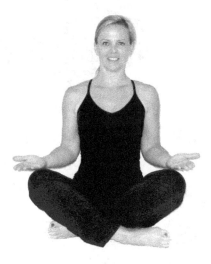 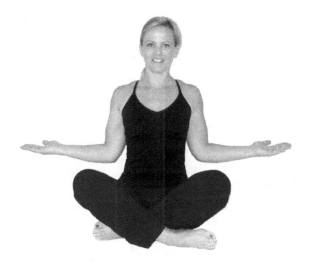

■Exhale as you serve the teacups to people on either side of you. ■Keep your elbows glued to your ribcage. ■Keep your armpits sliding toward your hips. ■Inhale as you bring your hands back to your starting position. ■Repeat 5x.

■**Notice** where you feel this movement. Some people feel a stretch in their chest, across the front of the shoulder, or along the back of the upper arm. Some people feel the muscles between their shoulder blades engaging.

■Note how far you can move without moving your elbows from your sides. Know that this **range of motion** will increase as you continue

Comfort Option: C
Comfortable Shoulders

Do you experience pinching sensations along the top of your shoulders? This is common when you've been driving or working on your computer for long periods? Dumbwaiter can help re-set muscle patterns that cause this sensation.

WINGS

Do this movement directly after Dumbwaiter. Wings helps you maintain shoulder blade mobility, while keeping your shoulders in your best Body Geometry This is a subtle movement that shows your body how to move your arms without over-using the top of the shoulder. Practicing this movement will ease tension in your neck and shoulders.

Begin this exercise sitting tall, kneeling, or standing. ■Glue your elbows to your ribcage and float your hands in front of you as if they were on a tabletop. ■Inhale as you scoop up the kittens, squeeze your seat and lengthen your spine.

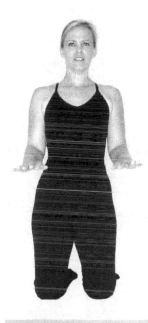

■Exhale to float your elbows up to the sides, like a pair of wings spreading out. ■Keep your armpits sliding low toward your hips. Your neck should feel long and loose. Take care to not allow your shoulders to ride up. ■Inhale as you return to your start position. ■Repeat 5x.

■**Notice** where you feel this movement. Hint: it's subtle. Your shoulder blades are rotating toward each other, like two disks on your back.

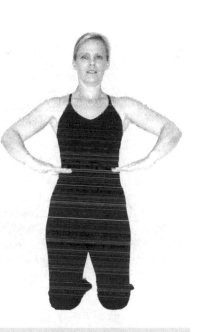

Body Geometry Boost: Try these Variations
- ■Try this movement with your palms facing up
- ■Try another Key Position: Cross Legged or Standing

LESSON 8: TABLETOP REACH

The Tabletop Reach lesson trains your body to support itself and move from the center *without laying down*. You'll tap into the strength of your powerhouse to hold up your torso and reach in different positions. As you extend your limbs outward, the challenge increases.

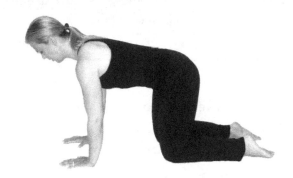

Anchor Points
for this Lesson

- **Baseline;** scoop in from hipbone to hipbone.
- **Ribcage;** knit the ribs inward, as if you were wearing a corset.
- **Hands, Feet & Shins:** lengthening the arms and legs, gently press the contact points — hands, feet and shins — into your mat. Ever so slightly, push the shin a tiny bit into your mat, as if you wanted to fully extend your leg.

Begin in Kneeling Tabletop 20-21

Scoop up the kittens to support your back. Inhale as you prepare for the movement.

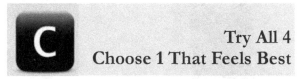

Try All 4
Choose 1 That Feels Best

- **Table Top Toe Reach**
- **Table Top Leg Reach**
- **Table Top Arm Reach**
- **Table Top Double Reach**

Illegal Movement Alert!
Your low-back & neck *must* remain relaxed during Tabletop Reach

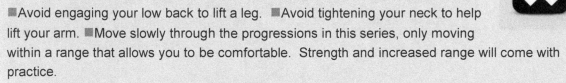

■Avoid engaging your low back to lift a leg. ■Avoid tightening your neck to help lift your arm. ■Move slowly through the progressions in this series, only moving within a range that allows you to be comfortable. Strength and increased range will come with practice.

Engaging the wrong muscles in this series will lead to overuse and can spiral into chronic tightness. When in doubt, have a friend lightly touch your low back or your neck as you perform the

TABLETOP REACH

Tabletop Reach activates the deep stabilizing muscles within your torso. The strong muscles of the hip work to raise the leg, while the arm begins its movement from your shoulder blade.

Table Top Toe Reach :
■Exhale as you extend your right leg back to straight, leaving your toes on the mat. Stretch the leg out, as if you wanted to grow an inch taller. ■Inhale as you return to your start position. ■Repeat 5x on each leg.

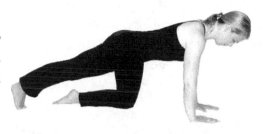

Table Top Leg Reach:
■Exhale as you extend your right leg back to straight, floating it up parallel to the floor. Extend the leg as long as possible. ■Inhale as you return to your start position. ■Now try this on your left leg. ■Repeat 5x for each side.

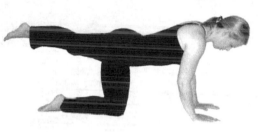

Table Top Arm Reach:
■Exhale as you float your right arm forward until it is parallel to the floor. Stretch the arm long **while pulling your shoulder away from your ear**. ■Inhale as you return to your start position. ■Now try this on your left arm. ■Repeat 5x for each side.

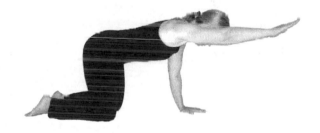

Table Top Full Reach:
■Exhale as you reach your right arm and left leg up, parallel with the floor. ■Keep reaching farther out while you scoop up the kittens. ■Inhale as you return to your start position. ■Now try this with the opposite arm and leg. ■Repeat 5x for each side.

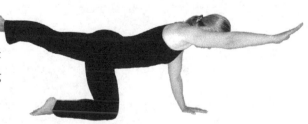

LESSON 9: LENGTHEN THE SPINE

The Lengthen the Spine lesson strengthens the long muscles on either side of your spine, as well as the back of your legs and hips. Always lengthen the spine first to create more space for the vertebrae, then gently float the breastbone up. The arch of the neck follows the arch of the spine. You may feel the rejuvenating effect that yogis have enjoyed for centuries via the practice of back bending.

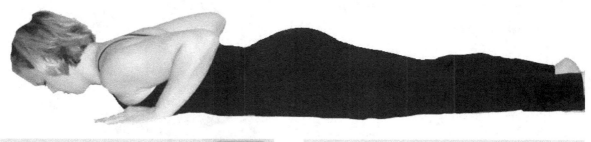

Choose 1 exercise

Begin in Prone Position 26

- Sphinx
- Cobra
- Dart

Anchor Points **for this Lesson**

- **Baseline;** scoop in from hipbone to hipbone.
- **Legs;** gently press them into your mat.
- **Armpits;** gently draw them toward your hips. Another way of thinking of this is to draw your shoulders away from your ears *without creating tension near the neck.*

- **Do not squeeze your Seat in this position.** Whenever you're considering arching the back even the tiniest bit, do not squeeze your seat, as it may cause undue tension in the low back.

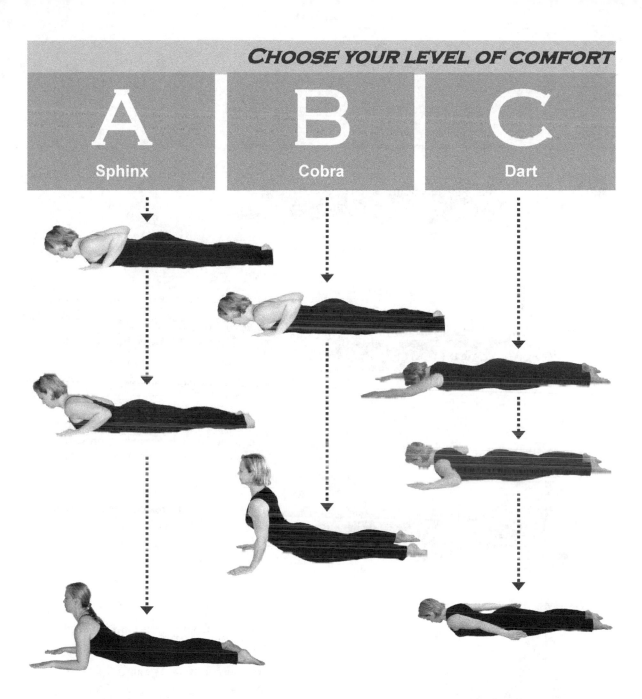

CHOOSE YOUR LEVEL OF COMFORT

A
Sphinx

B
Cobra

C
Dart

**Gently Float
the Breastbone Up**

**Continue Floating up
Until the Arms are
Fully Extended**

**Bend your Elbows
Toward Your Hips**

Then Extend the Arms

SPHINX & COBRA

So much of modern life encourages us to hunch forward — driving, cooking, working on a computer, etc. Sphinx and Cobra help reverse the effects of rounding forward by encouraging the spine to lengthen and arch. It feels like a breath of fresh air.

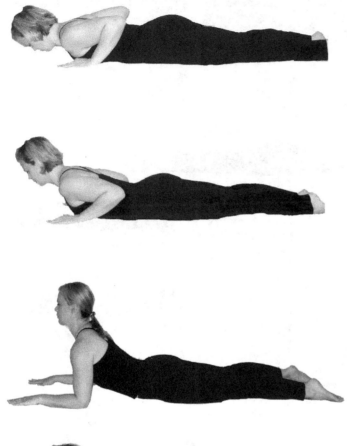

Begin in the **prone/face down position.**

Sphinx:
■Place your hands under your shoulders, drawing the shoulder blades down the back. **Create plenty of space between your shoulder and your earlobe.** ■ Press your palms and forearms into your mat. ■Draw the belly button in toward your spine, while keeping the legs active. Inhale to prepare to move.

■Exhale as you float your breastbone up and forward. Prop yourself up with your elbows under your shoulders.

■To make the arch more gentle on your spine, slide your elbows forward of your shoulders. ■Let your head balance easily on top of your spine. **Do not tilt the head back.**

Cobra:
Continue from your Sphinx position.
■Float the breast bone even higher, as you push into your palms. ■Some people will be able to extend their arms to straight. ■**Stay aware of how your back feels; choose your position based on comfort. You should feel no pressure in your low back.**

Repeat your preferred position 5x.

DART

Dart trains you to have good standing posture from the ribcage up. It opens your chest; sends your shoulders down and back; and lengthens the spine.

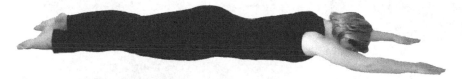

Begin **lying face down, arms extended forward.** Inhale as you scoop up the kittens.

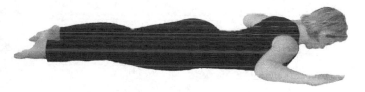

■Exhale as you lengthen your spine and lift your head and arms just off your mat. ■Your gaze should be only slightly lifted. **Lead with your breastbone**, not with your nose. ■Draw your elbows toward your ribcage while sliding shoulder blades down your back. ■Envision pushing water away with your arms; feel the muscles in your back engage.

■Keep sliding the arms back until your hands are by your hips. ■Feel your spine lengthening. Inhale to return to your start position.

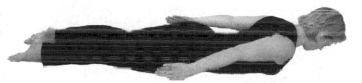

Repeat 5-10X

C Comfort Option: Sensitive Back today?

■Move only within your comfort range, focusing on lengthening the spine rather than arching it. Small, focused movements will help to ease any strain in your back; do not force anything!

Lifting your spine too high, too soon, can cause discomfort. ■**Make your range of motion small**, while lengthening your spine. As you create a little more space between each vertebrae, you'll gain the ability to arch more over time.

WORKOUT 3: MATWORK BASICS

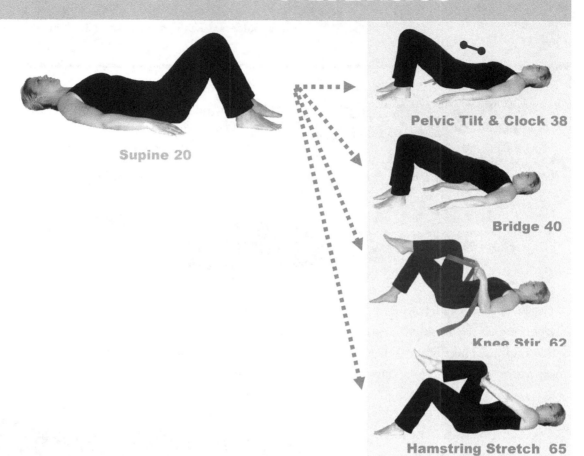

Supine 20

Pelvic Tilt & Clock 38

Bridge 40

Knee Stir 62

Hamstring Stretch 65

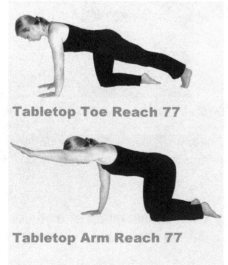

Tabletop Toe Reach 77

Tabletop Arm Reach 77

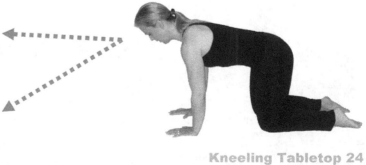

Kneeling Tabletop 24

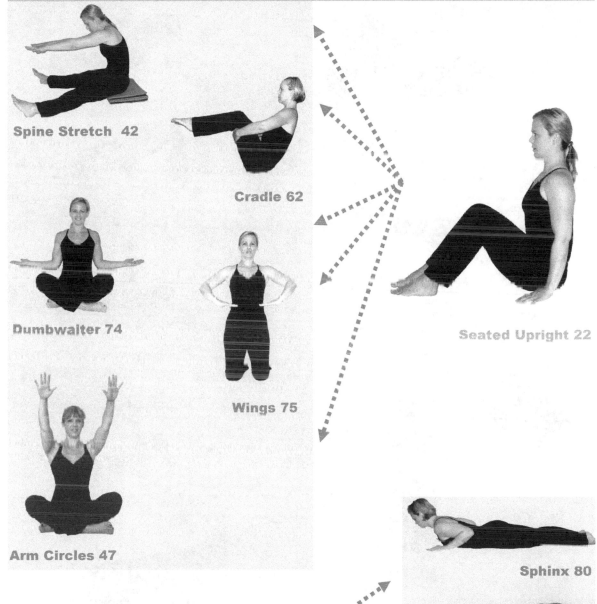

Spine Stretch 42

Cradle 62

Dumbwaiter 74

Wings 75

Arm Circles 47

Seated Upright 22

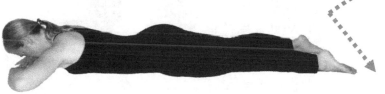

Sphinx 80

Childs Pose 35

Prone 26

WORKOUT 4: LONG & STRONG

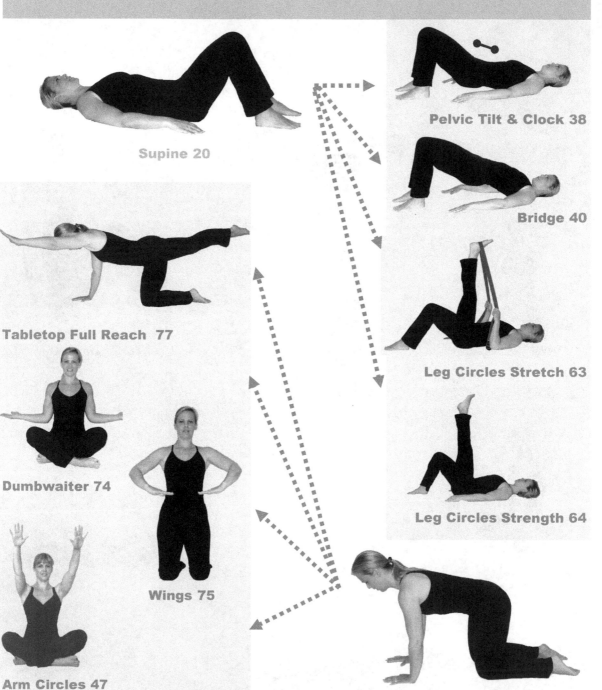

Supine 20

Pelvic Tilt & Clock 38

Bridge 40

Leg Circles Stretch 63

Leg Circles Strength 64

Tabletop Full Reach 77

Dumbwaiter 74

Wings 75

Arm Circles 47

Kneeling Tabletop 22

Perform each movement group 5x, before moving to the next group.
Work up to 10x Use the page numbers for instructions & anchor points.

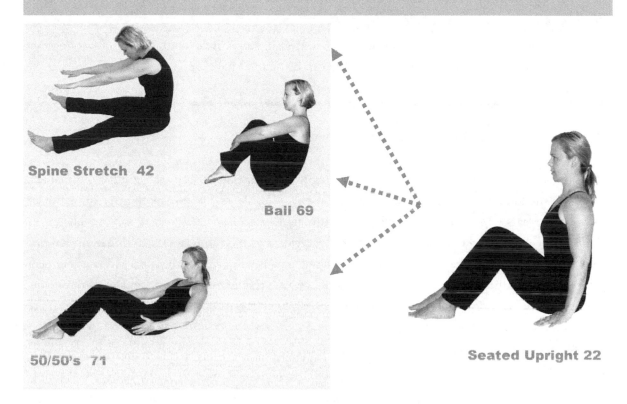

Spine Stretch 42

Ball 69

50/50's 71

Seated Upright 22

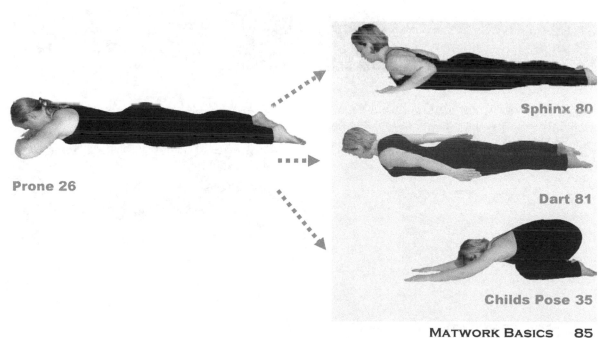

Prone 26

Sphinx 80

Dart 81

Childs Pose 35

WORKOUT 5: DRAWBRIDGE

This Drawbridge workout incorporates Roll Down, Bridge, Arm Circles, and Roll Up into one flowing series. Streaming these movements together can be quite a challenge. Give yourself a pat on the back for progressing this far!

Being in Sitting Upright Position. Hold onto the your thighs just above your knees.

■Inhale as you sit as tall as possible. Exhale during the movement. Push your feet into your mat and scoop up the kittens as you move into a **Roll Down.** ■Inhale as you float both arms up and back toward your ears. Move slowly, keeping your armpits low. ■Exhale as you float the tailbone up. Continue peeling one vertebrae at a time off the mat, to rise into **Bridge position**. Inhale as you prepare for the next movement. ■Exhale as you simultaneously lower your hips back down and slide your arms out to the sides. Envision pushing water away in this **Arm Circle** movement. ■When your hips touch the mat, move into a **Roll Up**, coming back to your start position.

Repeat 5-10x.

Body Geometry Boost: Add Light Hand weights

Try using small water bottles, or light hand weights to Drawbridge. Since shoulders can be sensitive, 3lbs maximum is plenty for women, 5lbs maximum for men.

Anchor Points for this Series

- **Baseline;** scoop in from hipbone to hipbone.
- **Ribcage;** knit the ribs inward, as if you were wearing a corset.
- **Seat;** squeeze your bottom.
- **Soles of your feet;** press these into the floor.

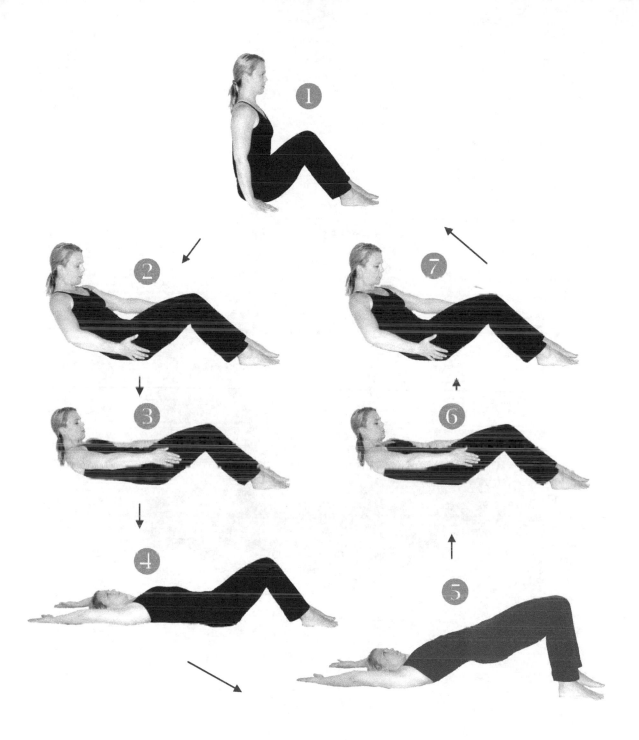

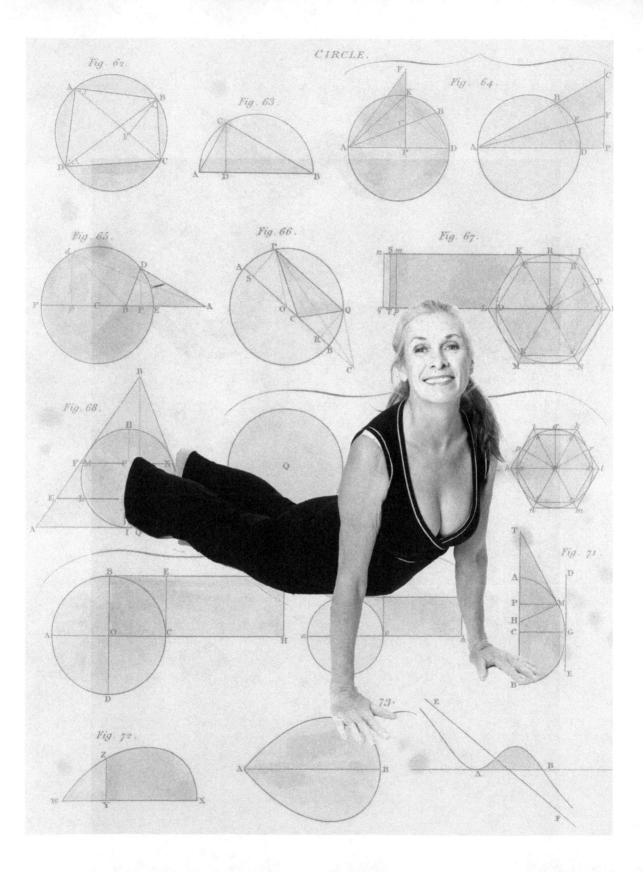

YOUR POWERHOUSE

Some say Joseph Pilates started the fitness trend of focusing on core strength. He coined the term **Powerhouse** when he wrote about strengthening the center of the body to support all of your movements. Think about how strong a ballerina or a fencer looks in their core as they perform precise and flexible movements with their legs and arms. This is the essence of the Pilates Powerhouse that we'll work on in the lesson.

LESSON 10: LOWER AB FOCUS

The Lower Ab lesson teaches you how to create a flat belly from the navel to the pubic bone. It activates both the abdominal muscles of the trunk and the hip flexor muscles that attach your leg to your torso. **Be sure to include one of the stretch options to keep your pelvis in balance**.

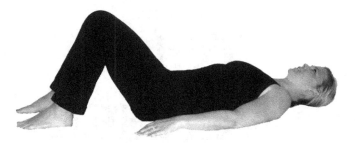

Try All 3 Exercises Choose 1

c

Begin in Supine/Knees Bent Position

- Knee Slides
- Toe Taps
- Single Leg Stretch

Body Geometry Tip:

Quiet your Torso

b

If this should become difficult:
- Check your **Anchor Points**;
- Make your **Range of Movement** smaller until you are able to stabilize your torso.

a

Anchor Points For this Lesson

Knees Bent

- **Baseline;** scoop in from hipbone to hipbone.
- **Seat:** squeeze your bottom.
- **Soles of your feet;** press these into the floor.

Legs Tabletop

- Baseline ■ Seat *and...*
- **Ribcage;** knit the ribs inward, as if you were wearing a corset.

CHOOSE YOUR LEVEL OF COMFORT

A
Knee Slides

B
Toe Taps

C
Single Leg Stretch

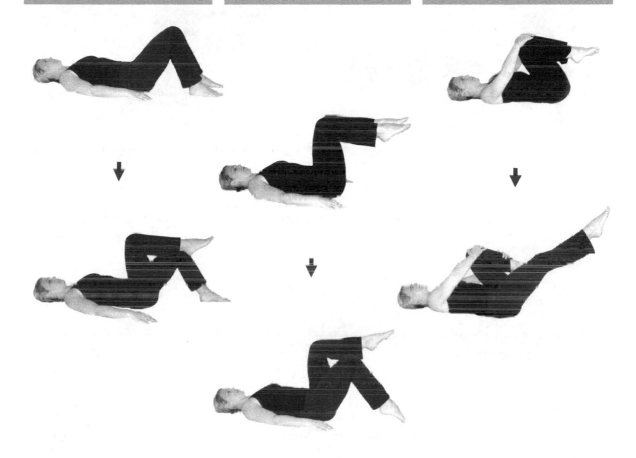

Float one knee toward The Sky

Move both Knees, Alternating One Up & One Down

Bicycle the Legs

KNEE SLIDES

Knee Slides activate the hip flexor muscles that lift your leg in every step you take. The stronger they are, the more comfortable you'll be when walking or running.

Begin in **supine, knees bent position**. Find your right hipbone with your right hand. Walk your fingers toward your navel 1-2 inches. Press in a bit with your fingertips throughout the following

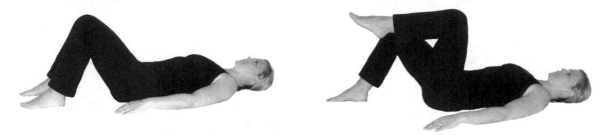

■Gently press your **left foot** down into your mat. Place your **left hand** on your **right knee**, use it to create resistance. ■Exhale as you scoop in the kittens and draw your right knee toward your shoulder. **Remember to resist the movement** by pushing with your left hand.

■Can you feel something under your fingertips? Some people feel a muscle become ropey, some people feel it flatten out a bit. These are your hip flexor muscles. Inhale to prepare for the next movement.

■Exhale as you push your right knee back to your start position, imagining you are pushing a great weight. Can you feel something working under your fingertips?

■Try the same movement on your left leg.
■Alternate legs, performing 10 knee slides on each leg.

Reclined Hip Flexor Stretch

Have a heavy pillow nearby to assist you in this stretch.

■From **supine, knees bent position,** slide one leg out long. ■Prop the pillow next to your foot so that your **toes point toward the sky**. (It will likely try to flop out to the side.) Your foot position is important for this subtle stretch. Don't use your muscles to maintain the position, use a prop of some sort. ■Breathe easily for 5-10 minutes, envisioning your low back relaxing into the floor. ■Switch legs, remembering to use the prop for your foot position.

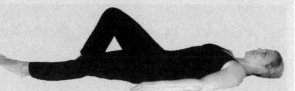

TOE TAPS

Toe Taps combine abdominal work with hip flexor work. You'll need to scoop more to keep your pelvis in neutral position. Remember your stretches afterward, to keep the body in balance.

Begin by laying down with your knees bent & feet flat on the floor. Scoop up the kittens, and float your knees up toward the sky. Inhale to prepare for the movement.

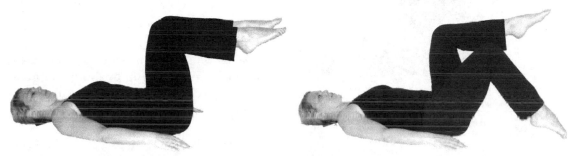

■Envision a **great weight just in front of** your **right foot**. ■Exhale as you push that great weight down toward the floor. Use your hip flexor, feel for it with your fingertips if you need to. Stop when your toes touch the floor, but don't rest your entire foot down. Inhale to prepare for the next movement.

■Envision a **great weight just in front of your right knee.** ■Exhale draw the right knee toward your shoulder, pushing that great weight. Use your hip flexor. Stop when your knee points toward the sky.

■Try the same movement on your left leg. ■Alternate legs, performing 10 toe taps on each leg.

Next Steps: ■Move both legs at the same time. Can you keep your pelvis in neutral while doing this? Moving both legs simultaneously is not a must.

Runner's Lunge Hip Flexor Stretch

b

Toe Taps are incredibly effective at strengthening and flattening the lower belly. Later in the day, when you move from sitting to standing, you may feel a strong pull where the leg attaches to the torso. This is your hip flexor stretching and flattening after your workout!

■Assist the stretch with a **kneeling lunge** to ease that pulling sensation.

SINGLE LEG STRETCH

Single Leg Stretch builds abdominal strength while stretching your legs and low back. I highly recommend this exercise first thing in the morning to get the blood pumping through your body. You'll feel energized and ready to jump into the rest of your day.

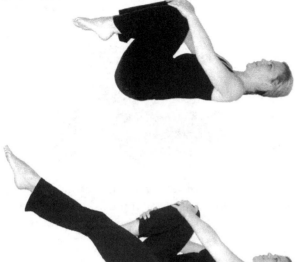

Begin in **Supine/Legs Tabletop position.** Activate your Anchor Points: **Baseline, Seat, Ribcage.** Inhale to prepare for the movement.

■Exhale as you push your right leg out to a 45-degree angle. **Envision pushing a great weight away with your foot.** Inhale to prepare for the next movement.

■Exhale as you switch the legs in a bicycling motion. ■**Continue to envision pushing a great weight with your foot when you push out, and with your knee when you pull in.** ■Scoop up the kittens; feel your hip flexors working.

Comfort Option: Choose an Appropriate Position

■**Notice:** Do you feel any discomfort in your low-back? If so, aim your leg higher up, you can even push your heel straight up to the sky if you need to.

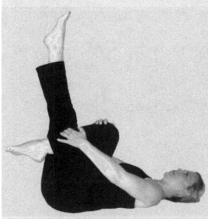

The lower your leg, the harder the exercise, the more potential stress on your low-back. ■**Choose an angle that feels like work on your abdominals, yet comfortable to your low-back.** Test out a new angle every few workouts.

Try the **Mini Roll-up** Position for Single Leg Stretch:

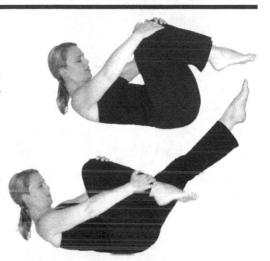

■Leading with your breast bone, lift your upper body as if you were beginning a **Roll-up.** Scoop and lift with the goal of peeling the top of your shoulder blade off your mat **Use your upper abdominals to power the movement.**

■**Tilt your gaze toward your knee**. ■Bicycle the legs. ■Envision pushing a great weight with your foot when you push out, and with your knee when you pull in. ■ Your goal is to keep your head up throughout the exercise, but if your neck begins to tire, put the head down.

Anchor Points **for the Tucked position**

- **Baseline;** scoop in from hipbone to hipbone.
- **Seat:** squeeze your bottom.
- **Ribcage;** knit the ribs inward, as if you were wearing a corset.

Illegal Movement Alert

The mini roll-up works the upper abdominals. When the abs begin to tire, your neck muscles will try to do the job. Since these tiny muscles are not built for this job, the neck becomes tired, stiff and sore. Whenever this happens, holding your head up has become an **Illegal Move**.

Body Geometry Tip: Checkpoints for this Position

While exercising in the mini roll-up position, aim to feel the bulk of the work happening just below your breastbone, where your ribs flare open. **This is new for most people, so expect these muscles to tire easily. That's ok!**

■**Check your Body Geometry;** is the gaze toward the knee; not toward the ceiling?
■**Check your Anchor Points:** are you corseting the ribs together? ■Begin the new position by **simply doing 1 or 2 repetitions** of your exercise with the head up, then continue with the head down. After a few sessions like this, try adding more repetitions with the head up.

LESSON 11: ARM & LEG COORDINATION

The Arm & Leg Coordination lesson shows you how to maintain a strong core while moving your arms and legs. Many people find that focusing on the core suddenly makes arm and leg movements stress-free. **When the body has an anchor, the extremities move with ease.**

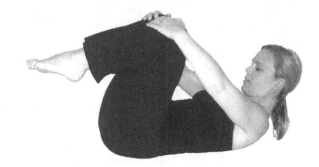

When the first Exercise becomes easy, move to the next

- **Table Top Arm Circles**
- **Double Leg Stretch**

Begin in Mini Roll-up/Tucked Position 21

Anchor Points for this Lesson

- **Baseline;** scoop in from hipbone to hipbone.
- **Seat:** squeeze your bottom.
- **Ribcage;** knit the ribs inward, as if you were wearing a corset.

Comfort Option:
Choosing your Position

While scooping up the kittens, allow the natural curve in your low back to occur. Try the Double Leg Stretch movement.

■**Does this cause tension in your low back?** If so, flatten the back all the way to the floor.

■**Does your back feel comfortable now?** If so, continue using this position for this exercise. If not, **it's too soon to do this exercise**.

■Perform Arm Circles with your natural low-back curve. Try Double Leg Stretch again in

A
Table Top Arm Circles

B
Double Leg Stretch

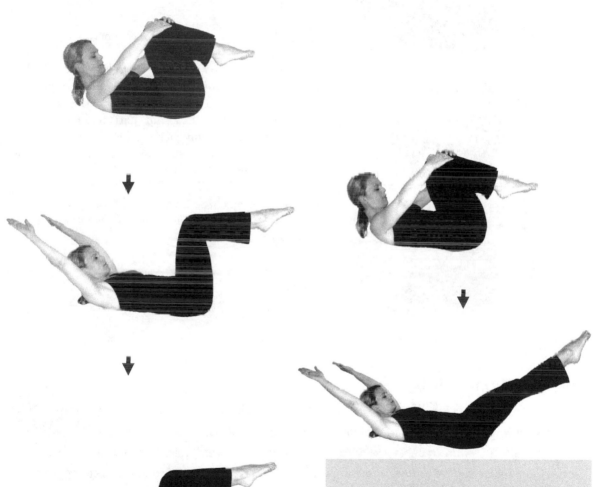

**Circle the Arms
While keeping Your Armpits Low**

Then, add a Leg Extension

TABLE TOP ARM CIRCLES

This exercise ups the ante by adding abdominal challenge to the arm circle movement. You're now working both ends of your powerhouse at the same time.

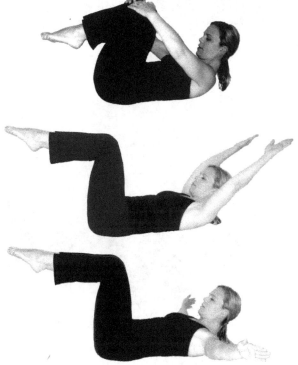

Begin in **Mini Roll-up/Tucked** position. Place your hands lightly on the sides of your knees. Scoop up the kittens as you move into a mini roll-up.

Inhale to prepare for the movement.

■Exhale as you float both arms up and back by your ears. **Move with control,** maintaining a low armpit. ■Inhale as you slide both arms out to the sides and around to your start position, as if you are swimming the back stroke. ■Envision pushing water away with your arms, this will engage your large back muscles.

■Mentally check in: are you keeping your armpits low? Are you keeping your pelvis in neutral position?

Repeat 10x

Comfort Option:
Getting into the Mini Roll-up Position Correctly

C

■**Lead with your breast bone, not with your nose.** This will activate your upper abdominals, instead of your neck. ■Your chin is tucked toward the notch at the top of your chest, as if you wanted to hold a tangerine there. ■Your shoulder blades are just beginning to peel up off the mat.

■**You can always alternate a few repetitions with your head up and a few with it down.** Your upper abdominals will become stronger as you continue to practice.

DOUBLE LEG STRETCH

Double Leg Stretch asks for even more core strength than your last movement. The big joint movements pump blood though the body, making you feel more alive. The arm and leg movements challenge both the abdominal and large back muscles. You're really working now!

Begin in **Mini Roll-up/Tucked** position. Place your hands lightly on the sides of your knees. Scoop up the kittens as you move into a mini roll-up position.

Inhale to prepare for the movement.

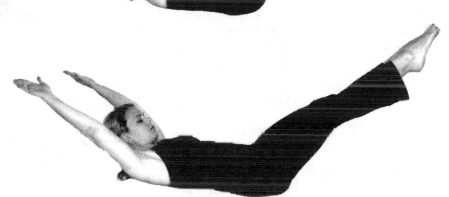

■Exhale as you push the legs out to 45 degrees and float both arms back by the ears. ■Keep your legs zipped together as if they are one unit. ■Inhale as you tuck the knees in to your center and circle your arms around to your start position. ■Use the image of pushing water with your arms and legs; this will activate more muscles.

Repeat 10x

■Mentally check in: are you keeping your armpits low? Are you keeping your pelvis in neutral position?

b **Body Geometry Tip:** Checkpoints for this movement
■Scoop up the Kittens
■Aim your legs higher than you think you need to; this will assist in keeping your torso quiet, or still.
■Gaze toward your legs, not toward the ceiling. This keeps the head in a balanced position; it will weigh heavily on the neck if you look skyward.
■Draw the armpits low to keep your energy focused toward the center of the body

LESSON 12: DOUBLE DUTY

This Double Duty lesson teaches you how to add heft to your ab work by supporting the weight of both legs during your movements. Always listen to your low back and adjust your position based on how your body feels each day. When performed without pain, these exercises will powerfully strengthen your mid-section, which is key to supporting your back.

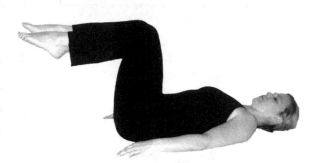

Do both of these Exercises

- **Double Knee Drops**
- **Double Straight Leg**

Begin in
Supine/Legs Tabletop Position 20

Body Geometry Tip:

Quiet your Torso throughout these movements

If this should become difficult:
■ Check your **Anchor Points**;
■ Make your **Range of Movement** smaller until you are able to stabilize your torso.

Anchor Points for this Lesson

- **Baseline;** scoop in from hipbone to hipbone.
- **Seat:** squeeze your bottom.
- **Ribcage;** knit the ribs inward, as if you were wearing a corset.

CHOOSE YOUR LEVEL OF COMFORT

A
Double Knee Drops

B
Double Straight leg

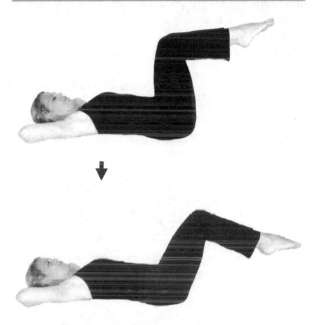

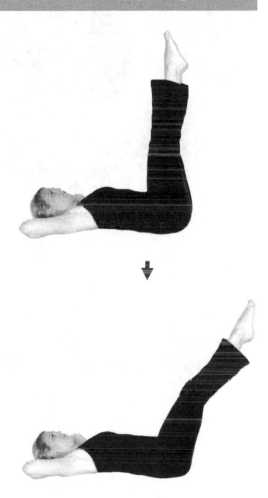

**Move from your Center Point
Move only the Legs**

DOUBLE KNEE DROP

Double Knee Drop strengthens your abdominals from the breast bone all the way to the pubic bone. Raising and lowering your bent legs works the mid and lower abdominals. Maintaining a mini roll-up position strengthens your upper abdominals.

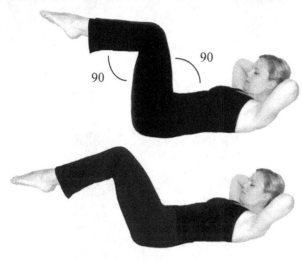

Begin in **Supine/Legs Tabletop** position. Cradle your head in your hands, using the arms to support the head. Scoop up the kittens as you move into a mini roll-up.

Inhale to prepare for the movement.

■Inhale as you float your knees forward. Aim to lower your knees until your toes just touch your mat, but stay aware of keeping your pelvis in neutral. ■Do not allow your lumbar curve to increase.

■Exhale as you scoop up the kittens a little harder, and bring your knees back up to 90/90.

Repeat 5-10x

■Aim to feel this exercise in your belly, not in your back. You can always choose to make your movement smaller.

Comfort Option: Be Aware of Neck Tension

If you begin to feel tension your neck, that's a sign that your upper abdominals are beginning to fatigue. ■Are you using your hands and arms to support the weight of your head? You can always rest your neck for a bit, while continuing the rest of the exercise. ■Try doing half of your repetitions with the head up and half with it down. On a good day, see if you can do more with the head up.

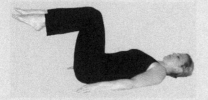 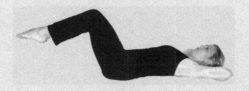

DOUBLE STRAIGHT LEG

The position of Double Straight Leg adds intensity to this movement pattern. A straight leg is more work for your body to move than a bent leg. . Choose this beefed up version when you're feeling strong, but remember that your torso needs to stay entirely still.

As **Double Knee Drop** becomes easier, lift your shins a bit higher, each day. One day, you'll realize that your legs are now vertical. ■It's ok to make your range of motion small as you experiment with extending your legs. ■Eventually, you will do this exercise with your legs extended fully. ■We call this **Double Straight Leg.**

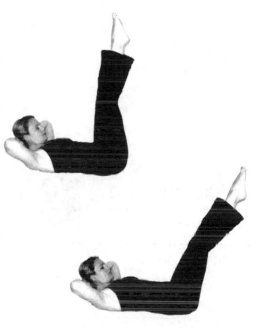

■Inhale as you float your extended legs forward. Make your movement very small, maybe 2 inches at first. ■Do not allow your lumbar curve to increase. ■Exhale as you scoop up the kittens a little harder, and bring your legs back up to your start position.

Repeat 5-10x

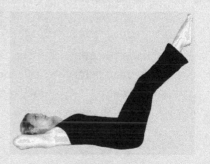

Comfort Option: Be Conservative with new Options

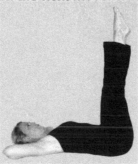

Whenever you move to a more challenging version of an exercise, make it as simple as possible. **You can always increase your Range of Motion (ROM) or lift your head on the next movement.**

LESSON 13: CORSET CINCH

The Corset Cinch lesson teaches you how to access all the muscles in your ribcage to create a corset of strength. Your torso will appear smaller and more tapered. More importantly, this corset aids you in standing upright with the posture of a fencer or a dancer. When your ribcage is engaged, there is no room to slouch.

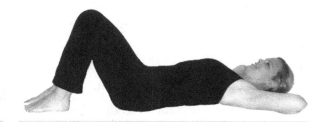

Try Both then Choose 1

Begin in Supine/Knees Bent Position 20

- Simple Criss Cross
- Criss Cross

Body Geometry Tip
Notice Your Efforts

Some movement patterns are **simple**, meaning 'not complicated.' This does not mean they are **easy. Give yourself credit for all of your hard work!**

Anchor Points for this Lesson

- **Baseline;** scoop in from hipbone to hipbone.
- **Seat:** squeeze your bottom.

CHOOSE YOUR LEVEL OF COMFORT

A
Simple Criss Cross

B
Criss Cross

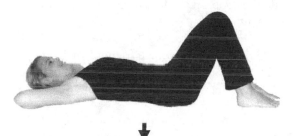

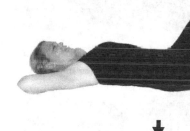

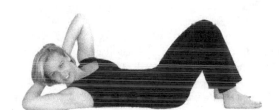

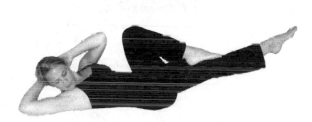

Keeping the lower body quiet,
Twist to Peel
your Shoulder Blade
Off the Mat

Add a Bicycling Movement
With the Legs

SIMPLE CRISS-CROSS

Simple Criss-cross is a fabulous method of building a natural girdle. You'll feel a new awareness of the muscles that knit your ribcage together and the work they do in supporting your upper body.

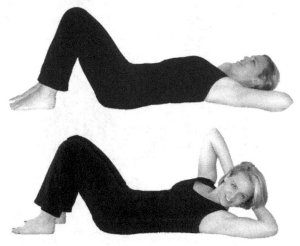

Begin in **Supine/Knees Bent position**. Cradle your head in your hands; elbows wide.

Inhale to scoop up the kittens and prepare for the movement.

■Exhale as you peel your left shoulder blade off your mat, keeping your elbows wide. ■Your goal is to twist so far that you can peek at your opposite elbow.

This is a big scooping and twisting movement. Keep your hips on your mat; allow your ribcage to swivel.

■Inhale as you come back to your start position. ■Pretend that someone is holding you up, and you need to work hard to roll down onto the mat. Put as much effort into this movement as you did into your first.

■Exhale as you peel your right shoulder blade off your mat, keeping your elbows wide. Inhale on the way back down.

Repeat 5-10x to each side.

Inefficient Movement Alert!
Momentum is _not_ your friend

Move slowly and deliberately, even when it seems like you've already completed the work phase of a movement. When you make every movement deliberate, you boost the effects of your exercise. 10 slow, precise criss-cross repetitions are always better than 50 quick, sloppy repetitions.

This compound movement combines Single Leg Stretch and Simple Criss Cross. Challenge yourself to perform it **slowly** and precisely.

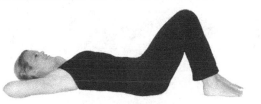

Begin in **Supine/Knees Bent position**. Cradle your head in your hands; elbows wide. Scoop up the kittens as you tuck your knees in to your chest.

Inhale to prepare for the movement.

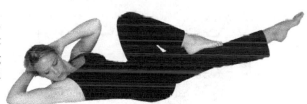

■**Exhale** as you push your right leg out to a 45% angle. At the same time, peel your right shoulder blade off the mat. ■Envision pushing a great weight away with your foot. ■Your goal is to peek at your opposite elbow.

■**Inhale** as you rotate your torso to center, and switch your legs. ■**Exhale** as you twist to the opposite side.

Alternate legs, performing 10 movements on each leg.

■Do not be concerned with touching the elbow to the knee, as this would be a very large Range of Motion. The largest ROM's come at the biggest cost: you must maintain a quiet torso from navel to public bone.

Comfort Option: Do you feel discomfort in your back?

If so, aim your leg higher up, you can even push your heel straight up to the sky if you need to.

■The lower your leg, the harder the exercise, the more potential stress on your low-back.
■Choose an angle that feels like work on your abdominals, yet comfortable to your low-back. ■ Test out a new angle every few workouts

WORKOUT 6: BUILD A POWERHOUSE

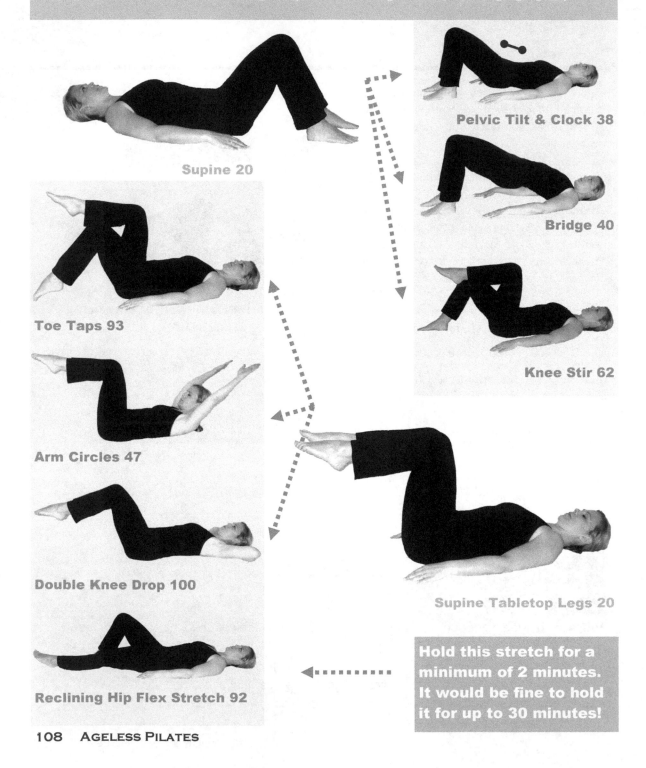

Supine 20

Pelvic Tilt & Clock 38

Bridge 40

Knee Stir 62

Toe Taps 93

Arm Circles 47

Double Knee Drop 100

Supine Tabletop Legs 20

Reclining Hip Flex Stretch 92

Hold this stretch for a minimum of 2 minutes. It would be fine to hold it for up to 30 minutes!

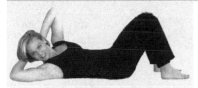

Simple Criss Cross 104

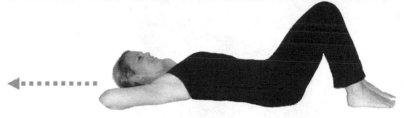

Supine 20

Wall Rollup 72

Press both feet entirely against the wall with toes slightly lower than your knees.

Press your hips into the floor and roll up one vertebra at a time.

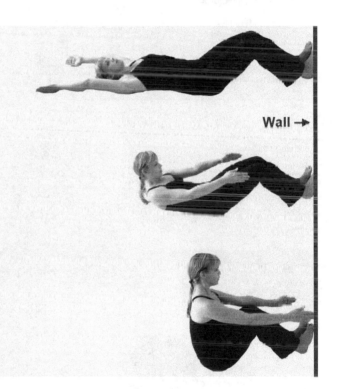

Wall →

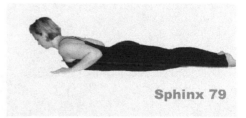

Sphinx 79

WORKOUT 6: WORKING THE POWERHOUSE

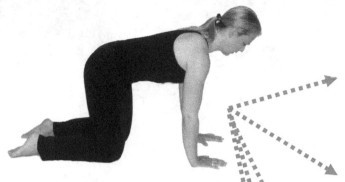

Kneeling Tabletop 24

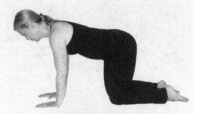

Pregnant Cat 32

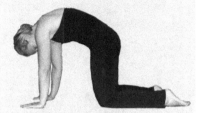

Cat 33

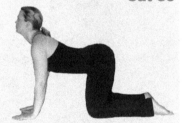

Cow 33

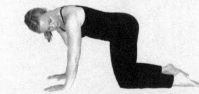

Dogtail 34

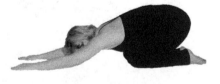

Child's Pose 34

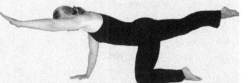

Tabletop Reach 77

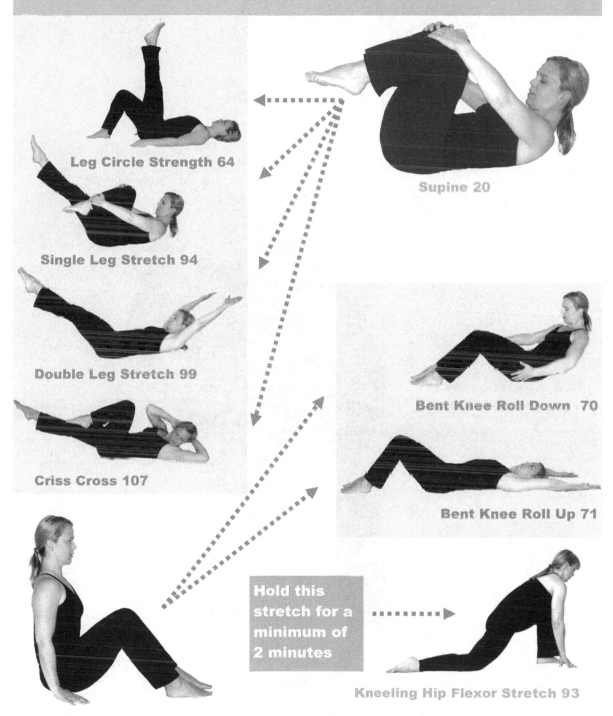

Perform each movement group 5x, before moving to the next group.
Work up to 10x Use the page numbers for instructions & anchor points.

Leg Circle Strength 64

Single Leg Stretch 94

Double Leg Stretch 99

Criss Cross 107

Supine 20

Bent Knee Roll Down 70

Bent Knee Roll Up 71

Hold this stretch for a minimum of 2 minutes

Kneeling Hip Flexor Stretch 93

Seated/Knees Bent 22

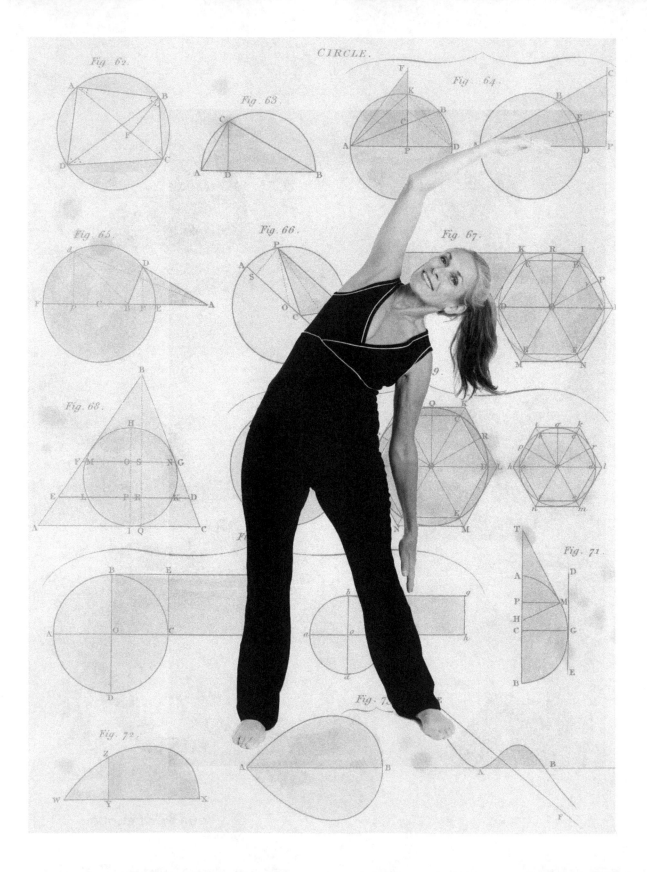

PERFECT POSTURE

Do you feel as if gravity is weighing you down? In this lesson, we'll learn how to change your body's relationship to gravity! When every body part is aligned relative to the whole, gravity supports you, rather than pulling at you.

You'll learn how to use your deep abdominals to move through all of the key spine positions — neutral, arched, flexed and side bend — increasing your strength and flexibility with every movement. **You'll feel gravity working with you, enhancing your energy.** Perfect posture is worth the effort.

LESSON 14: SIDE STRETCH

Side bending aids the health of your spine by encouraging the movement of fluid within your discs. Limber muscles in this area make your movements appear graceful.

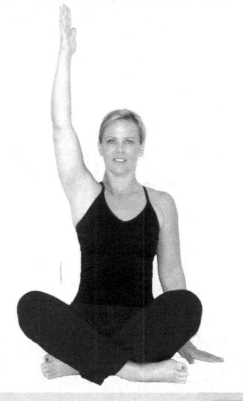

Choose 1   C

- Cross Leg Side Stretch
- Kneeling or Standing Side Stretch

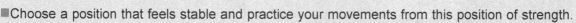

Comfort Option: Choosing Today's Position   C

Always honor the way your body feels right at this moment.

- Choose a position that feels stable and practice your movements from this position of strength.
- Every so often, try a new position to see if your stability options have increased. **Every day and every moment presents a new opportunity to choose** and a new opportunity to practice.

Side Stretch and Chest Expansion can be performed Seated in a chair, Cross-legged, Kneeling or Standing. **Choose the position that feels most stable to you today.**

A

Cross Leg Side Stretch

Arch to the Side

Keep the Spine Long

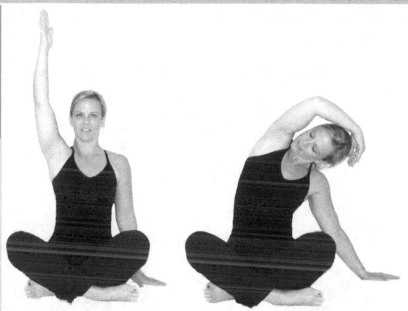

B

Kneeling Side Stretch

Arch to the Side

Maintain a Still, Quiet Pelvis

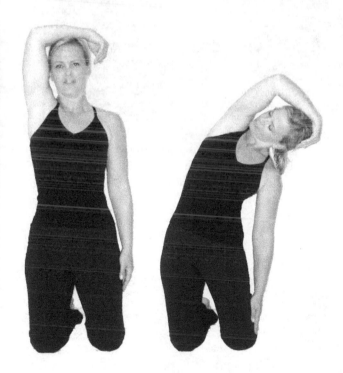

CROSS LEG SIDE STRETCH

Side Stretch lengthens the muscles that attach your torso to your hips. You'll feel longer, taller and more supple.

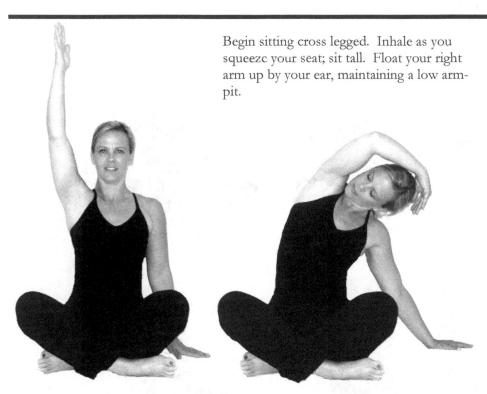

Begin sitting cross legged. Inhale as you squeeze your seat; sit tall. Float your right arm up by your ear, maintaining a low armpit.

■Exhale as you stretch to the left. Arch to the side as if you were rounding over an exercise ball. ■Allow the elbow to bend, wrapping your arm around your head. ■Feel the stretch on the muscles that connect at your armpit. Inhale as you return to center, bringing your arm down. ■Exhale as you stretch to the opposite side. Notice any differences from one side to the other. These will likely even out some over time.

Repeat 5x to each side.

Anchor Points **for this Lesson**

- **Baseline;** scoop in from hipbone to hipbone.
- **Seat;** squeeze your bottom.
- **Ribcage;** knit the ribs inward, as if you were wearing a corset.

KNEELING SIDE STRETCH

Kneeling Side Stretch requires more focus since you'll need to scoop even deeper to keep your hips still. You'll feel longer and taller as your core muscles separate your ribcage from your hips.

Comfort Option:
Fine Tuning

■Try this movement with and without a hand weight. ■Do you prefer the stretch that comes from adding a bit of weight to this position?

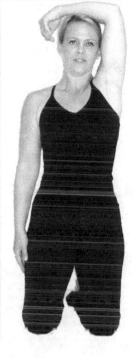
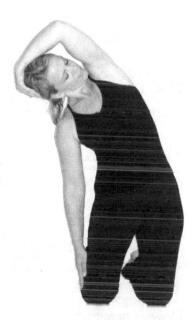

Envision your knees sinking into the ground, anchoring you down. Inhale as you lift your right arm up by your ear.

■Exhale as you arch to the left as if you were rounding over a barrel. ■Remember your **Box**; keep your hips level during this movement. ■Allow the elbow to bend, wrapping your arm around your head. ■Feel the stretch on the muscles that connect at your armpit. ■Feel the top of your buttock begin to stretch.
■Notice the placement of your dangling hand. Does it come close to your knee? Over time, your hand will reach farther down your leg. This is a sign that your range of motion is increasing. ■Inhale as you return to center, bringing your arm down.

■Exhale as you stretch to the opposite side.

Repeat 5x to each side.

LESSON 15: CHEST EXPANSION

The Chest Expansion lesson teaches you how to expand your lungs and release your neck tension. You'll notice a new ability to rotate your head farther. Your new range of motion will help you make safer lane changes while driving your car.

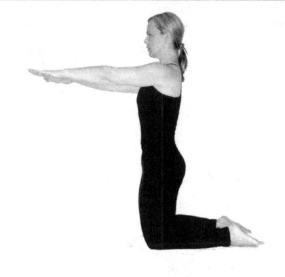

Choose 1

- **Chest Expansion**
- **Chest Expansion with Weights**

Comfort Option:
Choosing Today's Position

Always honor the way your body feels right at this moment. Choose a position that feels stable and practice your movements from this position of strength. Every so often, try a new position to see if your stability options have increased. **Every day and every moment presents a new opportunity to choose** and a new opportunity to practice.

Side Stretch and Chest Expansion can be performed Seated in a chair, Cross-legged, Kneeling or Standing. **Choose the position that feels most stable to you today.**

Anchor Points for this Lesson

- **Baseline;** scoop in from hipbone to hipbone.
- **Ribcage;** knit the ribs inward, as if you were wearing a corset.
- **Seat;** squeeze your bottom.

If Kneeling, add:

Feet & Shins: lengthening the legs, gently press the contact points — your feet and shins — into your mat. Ever so slightly, push the shin a tiny bit into your mat, as if you wanted to fully extend your leg. Feel how this encourages your body to lengthen upward.

A
Chest Expansion

Float the Arms Back

Armpit Stays Low As the Head Rotates

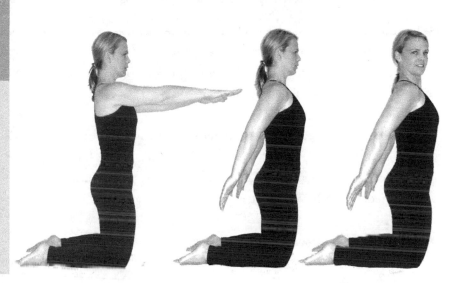

B
Chest Expansion
With Weights

Add Light Hand Weights

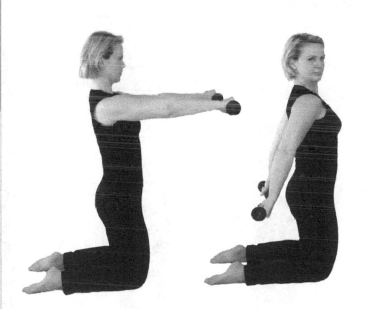

CHEST EXPANSION

Chest Expansion is excellent for easing forward shoulder slump. It draws your shoulder blades closer together while gently stretching your chest and releasing neck tension. The breathing pattern is famous for creating a sense of well being.

Begin in **Kneeling Upright** position. squeeze your seat, and sit as tall as possible. Inhale as you float both arms straight in front of you. ■To prepare for the movement, **exhale all air out of your lungs.** This will set up the full inhale to come.

■**Synch up your breath with your movement:** inhale as much air as possible while you press your arms down and back. Pretend you are pushing away water. ■**Hold your breath.** Slowly rotate your head to look over your left shoulder, turn back to center. Slowly rotate your head to look over your right shoulder, turn back to center.

■**Synch up your breath with your movement:** slowly exhale as you float your arms back up to your start position. Take the same amount of time for the breath and the movement; **exhale the last bit of air out of your lungs.**

Repeat 5x with head turns to each side.

■Note how far you can turn your head to each side. Can you rotate about the same amount to each side? Know that your range of motion will increase, and you will be able to turn your head farther and farther as you continue to practice.

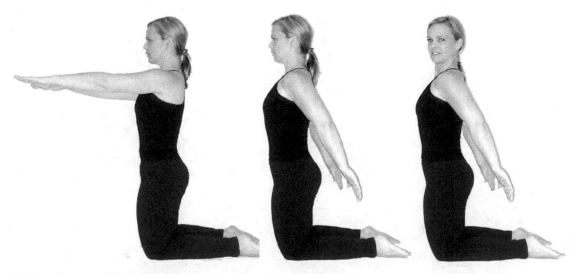

OPTIONS

Changing up your position from time to time stimulates different support muscles in the body, so that you're constantly working in new ways. This is good for both muscle and brain stimulation.

Add Hand Weights or Water Bottles(½ - 3lbs)

■This will help anchor down your shoulder girdle, and add to the stretch on neck muscles. ■There is no need to use a heavier weight.

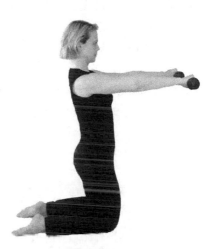

Cross Legged Chest Expansion

■Envision your sitting bones sinking down into the floor; this will help to anchor you throughout your movement. ■Take care to keep your weight evenly balanced on both sitting bones as you rotate your head.

Try Standing Chest Expansion

■Remember to lengthen toward both the ground and the sky. ■ Engage your **Seat** and your **Center Point** this will help anchor you. ■Only the head rotates, not the rest of the body.

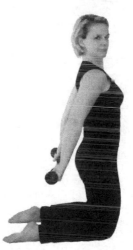

Body Geometry Tip:
This Breathing Lesson can lead to Euphoria

Don't rush through your breathing during Chest Expansion, or any Ageless Pilates movement.

Breathing deeply and slowly through your nose creates **nitric oxide**. This naturally occurring chemical opens your arteries, easing the blood flow to your heart and causing a mild euphoric sensation.

Since nitric oxide is a short-lived gas, the trick is to continue practicing this breathing method often.

LESSON 16: WORKING THE WALL

In this lesson, you'll use the wall as an anchor point while you work on posture enhancing exercises. Do these moves whenever you need to refresh yourself – after a long drive, on your coffee or lunch break or when you've been on your computer too long. When the body comes back into alignment, you'll feel so much better.

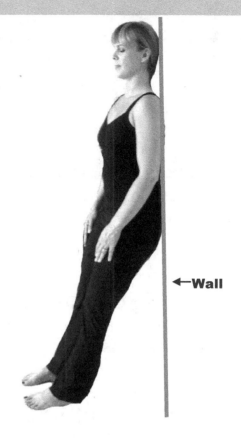

←**Wall**

Do All 3 of these Exercises

- **Wall Sits**
- **Wall Circles**
- **Wall Roll downs**

Anchor Points for this Lesson

- **Baseline;** scoop in from hipbone to hipbone.
- **Seat;** squeeze your bottom.
- **Ribcage;** knit the ribs inward, as if you were wearing a corset.

Begin in a Wall Lean

Lean your back against a wall, hinging at your hips so that your heels are about 18 inches from the wall. This will allow you to flatten your back against the wall. Scoop up the kittens, squeeze your seat, and push into your feet a little bit.

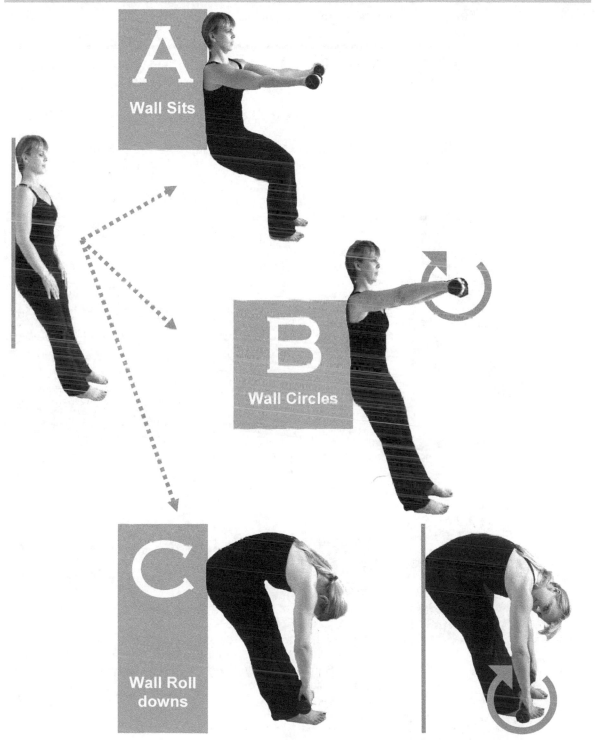

A
Wall Sits

B
Wall Circles

C
Wall Roll downs

WALL SITS

Wall Sits align all of the joints in your body while strengthening your thighs and hips.

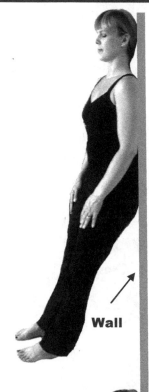

Wall

Begin in the Wall Lean position. Keeping your back flat against the wall, scoot your feet to 18 inches away from the wall.

Inhale to prepare for the movement.

Simultaneously: ■exhale, bending your knees to allow the hips to slide down the wall; ■float your arms up to shoulder height.

Simultaneously: ■inhale as you straighten your knees; ■float the arms back down to your sides.

Repeat 5x.

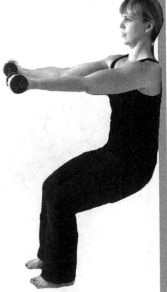

✖ Illegal Movement Alert!

■Don't allow your knees come farther forward than your toes.

■Don't allow your back to arch off of the wall.

■Are your knees locking when your legs are straight? Squeezing your seat will keep you from locking your knees.

b Body Geometry Boost

■Try Wall Sits, Circles and Roll downs with **small hand weights** (1/2 – 3lb) or holding water bottles.

■**Try Wall Sits with a bicep curl.** Instead of floating the arms to shoulder height, squeeze your bicep and bend at the elbow. Squeeze as if you were lifting a heavy weight, this will help to build a dense muscle.

WALL CIRCLES & ROLL DOWN

Wall Circles and Roll Down melt away neck and shoulder tension. Wall Circles heat the muscles, while the Roll down creates gentle traction on the neck and shoulders.

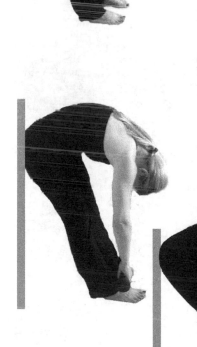

Begin with Wall Circles

Set up in the Wall Lean position. Hold light hand weights or small water bottles in your hands. Take a full inhale to prepare for the movement.

■Exhale as you draw large circles in front of you with both fists. This movement happens in the shoulder joint; **your arms stay straight.** Keep your hands within your vision. ■Synch up your exhalation and arm movement, so that they take the same amount of time. ■Inhale to prepare, exhale to move.

Repeat 5x in one direction, then 5x in the opposite direction.

Continue with a Roll down

■Drop your head, and slowly bring yourself into a passive hanging position. Peel one vertebra at a time off the wall, allowing your arms and head to dangle. ■Don't push to touch the floor, just hang passively.

■Slowly, draw 5 small circles about the size of a salad plate with your hand weights. Again, the movement happens in shoulder joint; the arms stay extended long. ■Draw 5 circles in the opposite direction as well.

■Slowly and gently, rotate your head as if you are saying no. Do this 5x.

■Let the head hang, scoop up the kittens a little harder, and roll back up to standing against the wall.

Don't skip the initial Arm Circles! This movement heats the muscles around the shoulders, which allows for a better release in the Roll down movement.

LESSON 17: SPINE EXTENSION

The Spine Extension Lesson continues our effort to create more space between every vertebrae. In this lesson, we'll add arm and leg movements at the same time, asking your body to tap into the proper muscles for each movement. When this happens, your back feels unburdened and effortless.

 Choose 1 That Feels Best

- **Single Leg Raise**
- **Letter X**
- **Swimming**

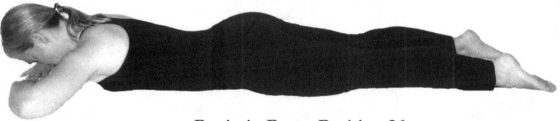

Begin in Prone Position 26

Anchor Points **for this Lesson**

- **Baseline;** scoop in from hipbone to hipbone.
- **Legs;** gently press them into your mat.
- **Armpits;** gently draw them toward your hips. Another way of thinking of this is to draw your shoulders away from your ears *without creating tension near the neck*.

Comfort Option: Be Kind to your Low-Back

- **Do not clench your Seat in this position.**
  Whenever you're considering arching your back even the tiniest bit, do not squeeze your seat with maximum intensity, as can cause tension in the low back. Squeeze just enough to activate your thigh muscles.

- **If you feel any discomfort in your low back**, you've lifted a little too high for your body right now. Make your range of motion a little bit smaller, and try to lengthen your spine more. As you create a little more space between each vertebrae, you'll gain the ability to arch more, over time.

A
Single Leg Raise

B
Letter X &Swimming

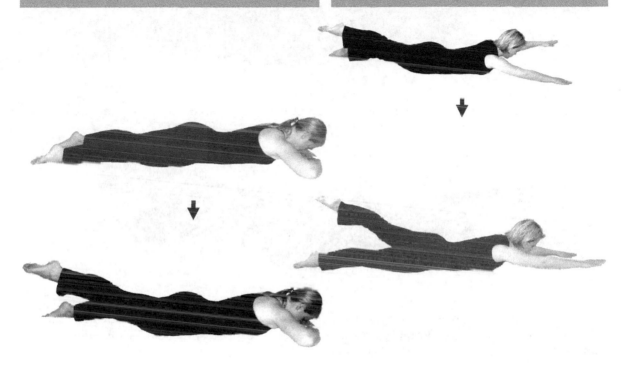

Anchor at the Baseline

**Lengthen the Leg
As you Lift it**

Anchor at the Baseline

**Lengthen Opposite
Arm & Leg
As you Lift them**

SINGLE LEG RAISE

Single Leg Raise encourages your seat and thigh to work together to lift your leg behind you. This movement pattern can eliminate low-back strain by teaching the body to use the correct muscles.

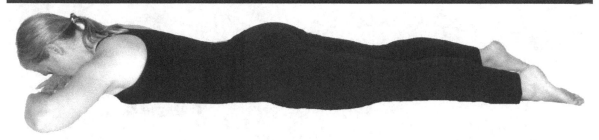

Begin in **Prone Position.** Scoop up the kittens and lengthen your spine to support and protect your low back. Inhale to prepare for the movement.

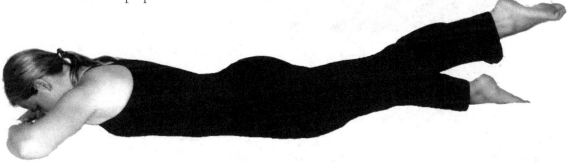

■Slowly exhale as you squeeze your seat and float your right leg up off the floor. Extend it as if you wanted to be an inch taller. ■Mind your low back,; don't reach farther up than feels comfortable. ■Draw out the time that it take to exhale. Inhale as you float the leg back down.

Repeat 5-8x on each leg.

Next Step: Try holding your lifted leg up through 2 full inhales and exhales

Illegal Movement Alert!
Focus on using the correct muscles to power this movement

■Mentally check in with your low back. ■It is cramped or uncomfortable in this movement? ■ Can you feel your low-back working to assist you, even if it is comfortable? ■If so, begin monitoring when this happens in your leg lift. Can you keep your back out of the exercise, if you limit your lift a bit? Avoid training your back to assist you in this movement, as it can lead to back and SI joint issues down the road.

LETTER X AND SWIMMING

Letter X adds an upper body lift to the Single Leg Raise. Your goal is to move both ends of the body without engaging your low-back.

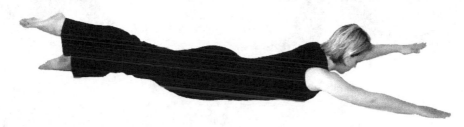

Begin in **Prone Position** with your arms and legs extended and separated. You should look like a capital letter X. Inhale as you scoop up the kittens and lengthen your spine.

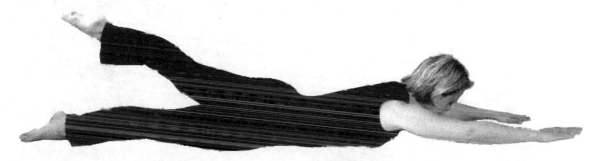

■Slowly exhale as you float your right arm and left leg up and out an inch. Lengthen your spine as you reach that extra inch. ■Mind your low back,; don't reach farther up than feels comfortable. ■Draw out the time that it take to exhale. Inhale as you return to the mat.

Repeat 5-8x on each arm/leg.

Body Geometry Boost: Your Next Step

Kick it Up with Swimming   Begin in Letter X position, lift your head up to look forward. Instead of holding your Letter X position, quickly move the arms and legs, simulating a crawling swim stroke.

- Draw the belly button up toward your spine
- Lengthen the spine and the torso
- Draw out the time it takes to inhale & exhale

WORKOUT 8: LENGTHEN & STRENGTHEN

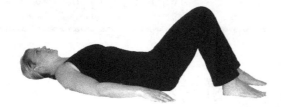

Supine 20

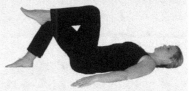

Knee Stir 62

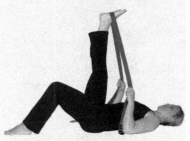

Leg Circle Stretch 63

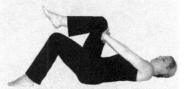

Hamstring Stretch 65

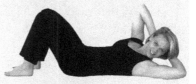

Simple Criss Cross 106

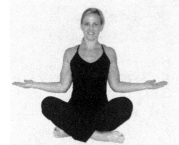

Dumbwaiter 74

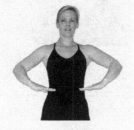

Wings 75

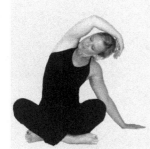

Side Stretch 116

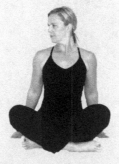

Chest Expansion 120

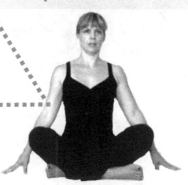

Seated Cross Leg 23

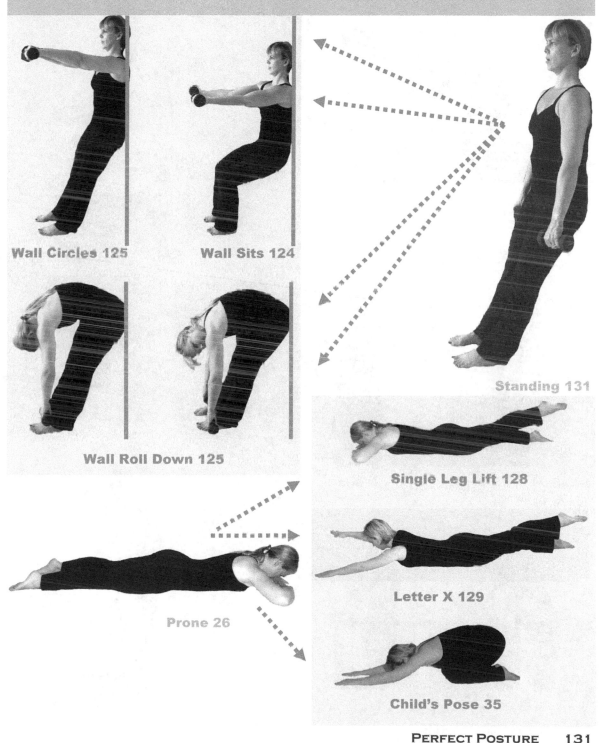

Perform each movement group 5x, before moving to the next group.
Work up to 10x Use the page numbers for instructions & anchor points.

Wall Circles 125

Wall Sits 124

Wall Roll Down 125

Standing 131

Single Leg Lift 128

Letter X 129

Prone 26

Child's Pose 35

WORKOUT 9: FEELING TALL

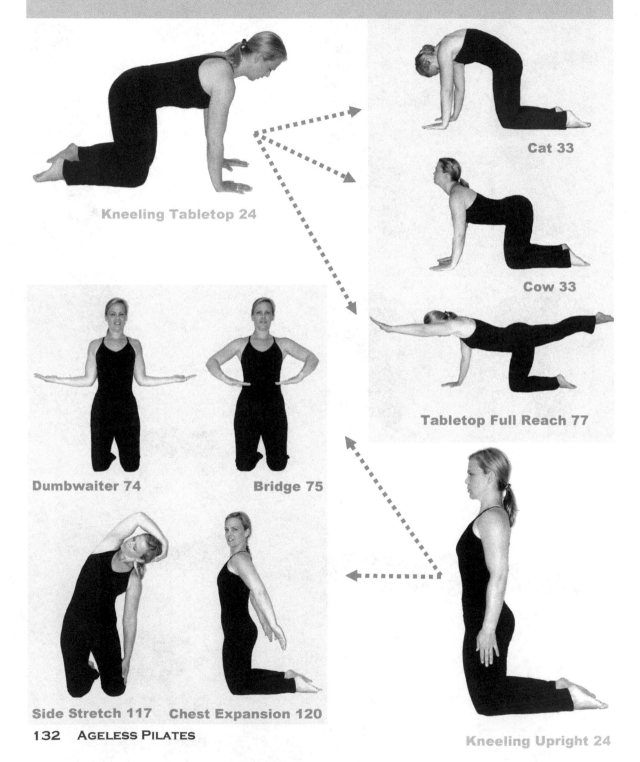

Kneeling Tabletop 24

Cat 33

Cow 33

Tabletop Full Reach 77

Dumbwaiter 74

Bridge 75

Side Stretch 117

Chest Expansion 120

Kneeling Upright 24

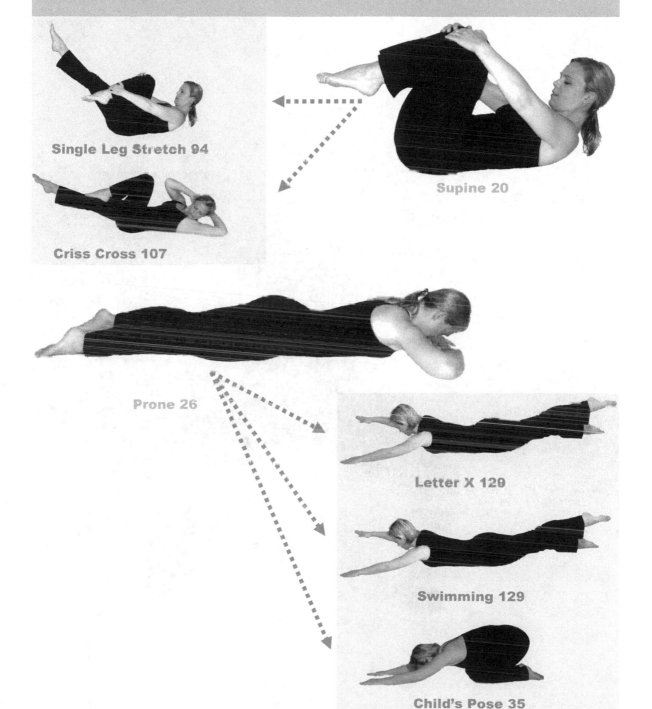

Perform each movement group 5x, before moving to the next group.
Work up to 10x Use the page numbers for instructions & anchor points.

Single Leg Stretch 94

Criss Cross 107

Supine 20

Prone 26

Letter X 129

Swimming 129

Child's Pose 35

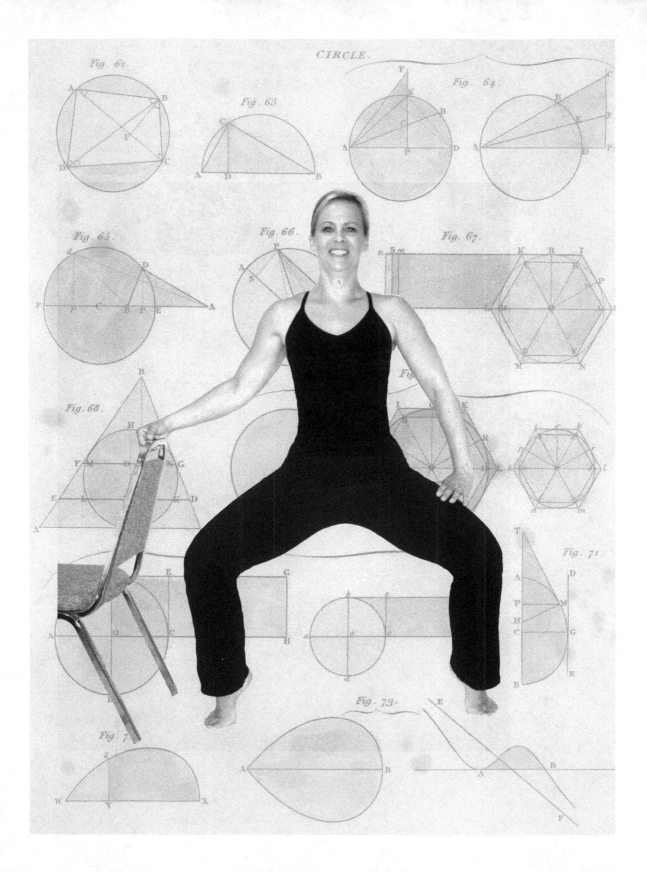

BALANCE BUILDERS

When you notice the grace in a ballerina or fencer's movements, you're noticing their ability to balance and move within the forces of gravity. It's an essential life skill for walking, running, golfing, you name it. We use it to preventing falls and fractures over the course of a lifetime. This chapter spans from basic balance builders to moves that will help you fine-tune your fluidity. The new elongated physique you'll build is a fine side benefit.

LESSON 18: KNEELING LUNGE

The Kneeling Lunge Lesson works on balancing out both sides of your hip and thigh musculature. When one hip or thigh is tighter or stronger, it throws off your standing balance.

This kneeling position allows you to work on stretching the hip flexors in your back leg as you strengthen the thigh of your front leg. This combination will have you feeling light on your feet in no time.

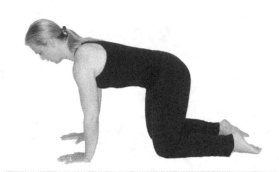

Begin in Kneeling Tabletop 24

Choose 1 That Feels Best

- **Kneeling Lunge**
- **Upright Kneeling Lunge**
- **Extended Kneeling Lunge**

Anchor Points **for this Lesson**

a

- **Baseline;** scoop in from hipbone to hipbone.
- **Ribcage;** knit the ribs inward, as if you were wearing a corset.
- **Seat:** squeeze your bottom.
- **Hands, Feet & Shins:** lengthening the arms and legs, gently press the contact points — hands, feet and shins — into your mat. Ever so slightly, push the shin a tiny bit into your mat, as if you wanted to fully extend your leg.

Kneeling Lunge

Begin in **Kneeling Tabletop position**. Inhale as you prepare for the movement. ■Exhale, as you lift up your right knee and draw the right foot between your hands. ■Scoop up the kittens to initiate the movement of your leg. ■Take 2-3 slow breaths in this position as you fine tune yourself.

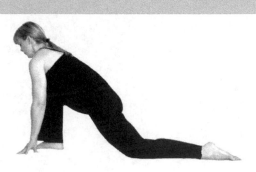

KNEELING LUNGE

In the three versions of Kneeling Lunges, your stretch increases as you move from a low position to a higher one. Your hip flexors stretch in each position. As you come to upright, the muscles in your torso stretch and flatten. Reaching the arms overhead lengthens the side and back of the torso.

Upright Kneeling Lunge

■From your Kneeling Lunge position, place your hands on your upright knee, pushing yourself into to an upright position. ■Continue to scoop up the kittens. Lengthen your spine as much as possible. ■Take a few slow breaths in this position.

■Run through your fine tuning list again, as the body has a way of shifting when we add a new challenge.

■Return to **Kneeling Tabletop** position. Repeat with your left leg forward.

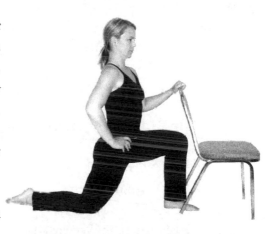

Body Geometry Tip: Fine Tune Your Position
■Level out your hips. ■Push into your right foot so that you can stabilize with your right leg ■Drop forward with your left hip bone. ■Feel your left hip stretching. ■Feel your upright leg working

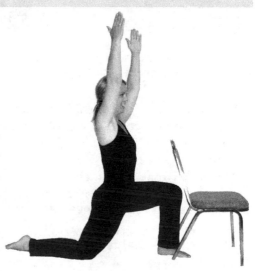

Extended Kneeling Lunge

■From **Upright Kneeling Lunge position**, raise the left arm high in the air, keeping your armpit low. ■Try raising the right arm up as well, so that both hands are reaching for the sky. ■Lengthen the spine. ■Try shifting your gaze up toward the sky.

■Run through your fine tuning list.

LESSON 19: STANDING BALANCE

This Standing Balance Lesson can help you assess if one leg has become stronger than the other. A strength difference over time can cause tension that throws off your balance. Try doing these exercises in front of a mirror so that you can see your hip bones and manage your Body Geometry.

Do Both Movements

- **Standing Knee Lifts**
- **Standing Leg Lifts**

Begin Standing Upright

If you feel the need, place one hand on a nearby chair or table.

Comfort Option:

Do these exercises throw you off balance?

You can work on them in a seated Position (photos on p.148)

- Sit in a chair, with both feet flat on the floor. Inhale, scoop up the kittens and sit tall.

- As you exhale, float one knee several inches up. Your foot will be off the floor. Inhale as you float the knee back down.

- Try holding the leg up for three full breaths.

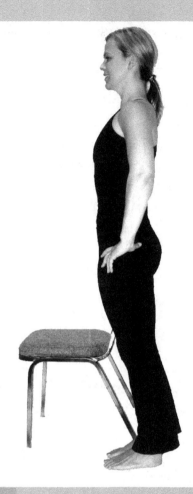

Anchor Points for this Lesson

- **Baseline;** scoop in from hipbone to hipbone.
- **Ribcage;** knit the ribs inward, as if you were wearing a corset.
- **Seat:** squeeze your bottom.
- **Soles of your feet;** press these into the floor.

STANDING LIFTS

This movement pattern helps your body differentiate between the muscles that stabilize the center of your body, and the muscles that lift your leg comfortably. Your ability to comfortably lift your leg affects your comfort in walking and moving in daily life.

Begin in the **Standing Upright** position. Inhale as you prepare for the movement.

Standing Knee Lifts

■Shift your weight onto your left foot. ■Exhale as you float your right knee up, bringing your foot off the floor. ■Float to wherever you feel comfortable balancing. This may mean lifting your knee so that just your toes are touching the floor. Or, it may mean that you can lift your knee until it is level with your waist.

■Inhale as you float the knee back down, placing your foot solidly on the floor ■Repeat on 5x on each leg.

Standing Leg Lifts

■Try the same pattern with a straight leg. The leg will feel as if it weighs more, so don't expect the movement to be as large.

Next Step:

■Try holding the lifted knee for three inhales and exhales. ■Do this at whatever level you are lifting your knee; it will help to build your stamina. ■Next time, try lifting your leg a tiny bit higher.

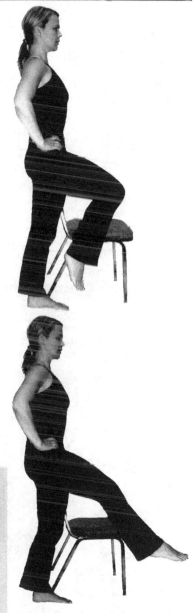

Body Geometry Check Your Box

Don't guess, use a mirror! ■**Are your shoulders level and centered over your hips?** Your body may be compensating by shifting your weight. ■Try drawing your armpits toward your hips. ■**Are your hips level?** When the seat is weaker on one side, it often causes your low-back to engage on the opposite side. This will send your hips off-kilter when you're standing on one leg. ■Try lowering your leg a bit so that you can level them out.

LESSON 20: STANDING LUNGE

Have you ever seen the lunge of a graceful fencer? It's a beautiful sport to watch. Lunges are the hallmark of fencers training, as they stretch and strengthen each leg independently. You'll notice a new gracefulness and a renewed sense of balance in your stride.

Try All 3

- **Forward Lunge**
- **Backward Lunge**
- **V-Lunge**

Begin Standing Upright 20-21

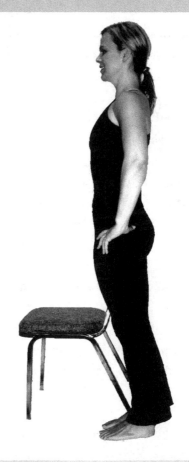

Anchor Points for this Lesson

- **Baseline;** scoop in from hipbone to hipbone.
- **Ribcage;** knit the ribs inward, as if you were wearing a corset.
- **Seat:** squeeze your bottom.
- **Soles of your feet;** press these into the floor.

Comfort Option:
Stay Steady, Use a Prop

- Perform these moves next to a sofa, table or study chair, so that you can reach out to steady yourself if needed. It's ok to begin holding on, then try letting go.

- **Notice** whether your body feels different from one side to the other.

CHOOSE YOUR LEVEL OF COMFORT

A	B	C
Forward Lunge	**Backward Lunge**	**V-Lunge**
Step Forward Allow the knees to bend comfortably	Step Backward Allow the knees to bend comfortably	Step on a Diagonal Allow the front knee to bend comfortably

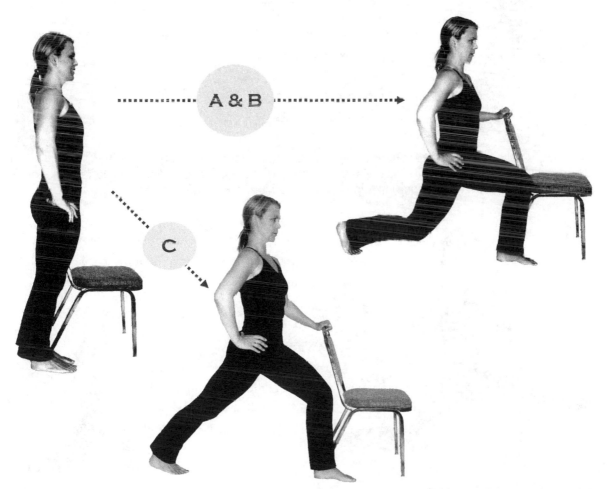

A & B

C

Forward & Backward Lunge

Lunges build your balance skills while strengthening your thigh and hips. You may find that you have more spring in your step as you continue to practice.

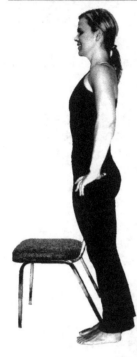

Begin in the **Standing Upright** position. If you are using a piece of furniture to steady yourself, line up your left hip alongside it. Inhale as you prepare for the movement.

Forward Lunge

■Exhale as you step forward with your right foot. ■Allow both knees to bend comfortably; choose your range of motion based on your comfort. ■ Bend your right knee so that it floats over the top of your right foot. ■Take 2 -3 slow breaths in this position as you fine tune yourself

■Return to your start position. ■Now try a Standing Lunge with your left leg forward. ■Repeat 5x on each leg.

Body Geometry Tip:
Fine Tune your Position

b

■Level out your hips. ■Push into your right foot so that you can stabilize with your right leg. ■Drop forward with your left hip bone. ■ Feel your left thigh & hip stretching. ■Feel your upright leg working

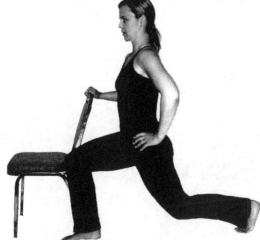

Backward Lunge

■Adjust your step to be **backward.** ■Move slowly, as the change in direction may be more challenging than you anticipate. ■Use your Fine Tuning List.

Arm Raises

■When your right leg is forward, try raising the left arm. This will accentuate the stretch on the leg. ■ Raising both arms earns you a bonus point for balance

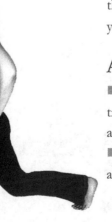

V-Lunge & Fencer's Lunge

V-Lunge and Fencer's Lunge train your body to be comfortable stepping out at angle,. This is so handy when you need to avoid a bump in the sidewalk or something inadvertently left in your path.

Begin in the **Standing Upright** position.

V-Lunge:
■Exhale as you step **diagonally to the right** with your right foot. ■Keep your left leg straight. ■Bend your right knee so that it floats over the top of your right foot.. ■Take 2-3 slow breaths in this position as you fine tune yourself

■Return to your start position. ■Now try a V-Lunge with your left leg forward. ■Repeat 5x on each leg.

Fencer's Lunge:
■As you step to the right, extend your left arm diagonally up as well, as if you were reaching forward with a sword. ■Feel the stretch expand along your left side, from the hand, through the torso, and along the leg.

■Switch arms when you switch legs. ■The extended arm matches up with the straight, extended leg.

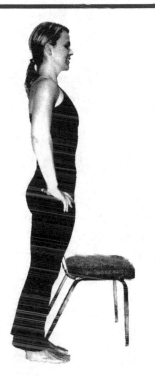

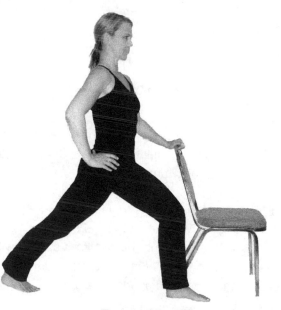

b Body Geometry Tip:
Keep your Eye on the Prize

■Be like the fencer who looks forward, at his opponent. ■Whether you're walking down the street or you're lunging in place, direct your gaze forward. Looking at your feet will not improve your balance. If you feel unsteady, simply hold onto something while you're lunging.

Plies are the cornerstone of ballet training, strengthening and stretching your hips and bottom in ways that you may have forgotten. Many people find that loosening the hips alleviates low back pain by opening and releasing the sacroiliac joint.

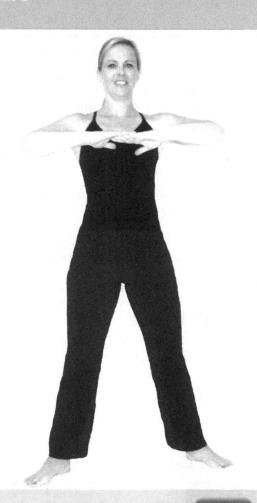

Begin Standing in Wide Pilates V

25

Stand upright in Pilates V position, heels touching, toes apart. Scoop up the kittens, lengthen your spine and squeeze your seat. Now step to the side so that your feet are slightly past shoulder width.

Try All 3

- Basic Wide Plie
- Heel Lifts
- Plie Curls

Comfort Options:

■Deep plies are Not necessary
Simply bend and extend the ankle, knee and hip joints at the same time. You'll be on your way to pumping lymph — life enhancing fluids — through your system while gaining strength, flexibility and balance.

■Build your Foot Muscles by going Shoeless
Try your plies without shoes. Is there a difference in your ability to balance and move? Orthotics can be helpful in daily life, but they will not retrain the support muscles in your foot. When standing, gently push through your heel and the base of the big and little toes. Activate your arch by pretending to dome it up a bit.

C

WIDE PLIE OPTIONS

Wide plies tone your hips and thighs. By using good Body Geometry, you'll also tone the muscles of your feet , which are key to maintaining good balance throughout your life.

Begin standing in **Wide Pilates V** position. Inhale as you scoop up the kittens, lengthen your spine and prepare for the movement.

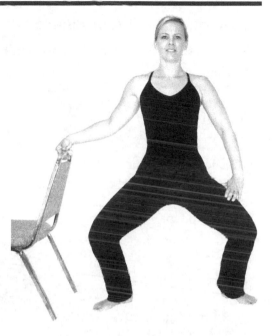

Basic Wide Plie

■Exhale as you squeeze your seat and bend your knees to lower into a plie. Keep your heels down; **simply lower comfortably** without losing your balance. ■Inhale as you raise up to your start position.

Heel Lifts/Part 1

■Lower into your plie position. ■Lift your heels off the floor slightly. ■**Keeping your heels up**, extend the legs to straight. ■Lower your heels to the floor with control.

Heel Lifts/Part 2

■From standing, lift your heels slightly off the floor. ■**Keeping your heels up**, lower into a plie. ■In your low position, place your heels down with control. ■Return to **Wide Pilates V** position.

Plie Curls

■Hold light hand weights (1/2 – 3 lbs) or water bottles in each hand, palms facing forward. ■As you bend your knees to plie, bend your elbows. ■Keep your elbows glued to your ribcage, and squeeze your bicep as you move the arm. ■As you straighten your knees, straighten your arms.

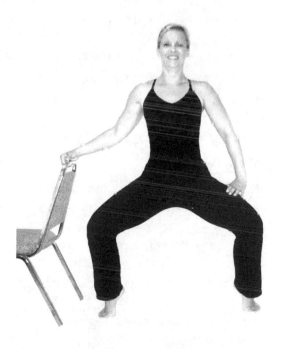

■Try this move with your palms facing each other as well. ■Doing this exercise with two different hand positions creates a stronger, shapelier arm.

For each movement: try 5x today, work up to 10x.

LESSON 22: NARROW PLIES

Begin Standing in Pilates V

Stand upright in Pilates V position, heels touching, toes apart.

Try All 3

- Basic Narrow Plie
- Heel Lifts
- Plie Zip Ups

Anchor Points
for this Lesson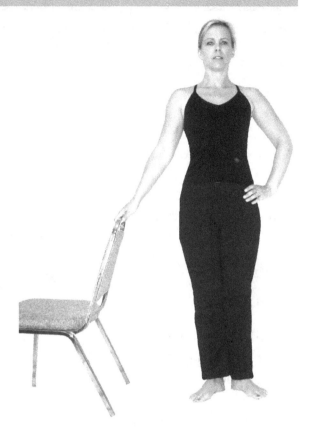

- **Baseline;** scoop in from hipbone to hipbone.
- **Ribcage;** knit the ribs inward, as if you were wearing a corset.
- **Seat:** squeeze your bottom.
- **Soles of your feet;** press these into the floor.

Body Geometry Tip:
Why is a Narrow Plie more difficult than a Wide Plie?

It's not your imagination, this is a more difficult position! In fact, it's very likely that you will not be able to drop as low as when doing a Wide Plie.

Bringing your heels together narrows your base of stability, making balance more difficult. If this position proves to be too much, try lightly holding a nearby chair or sofa. It's also ok to separate your heels slightly until you can stand comfortably.

Tip: keeping the heels touching is a function of creating an anchor point at your seat. **Squeeze the seat,** and it will be much easier to keep your heels together.

NARROW PLIE OPTIONS

Narrow plies add a balance challenge to the toning work of the wide plie. Squeeze your seat, keep your joints lined up, and you'll see amazing improvement in your walking gait.

Basic Narrow Plie

■Exhale as you squeeze your seat and bend your knees to lower into a plie. ■Keep the **heels touching together.** ■Keep the **heels down**, simply lower as much as you can without losing your balance. ■Inhale as you raise up to your start position. ■ Repeat 5x today, work up to 10x.

Heel Lifts/Part 1

■Lower into your plie position. ■Lift your heels off the floor slightly. ■**Keeping your heels up**, extend the legs to straight. ■ Lower your heels to the floor with control.

Heel Lifts/Part 2

■From standing, lift your heels slightly off the floor. ■**Keeping your heels up**, lower into a plie. ■In your low position, place your heels down with control. ■Return to **Standing Pilates V** position.

Plie Zip Ups

■Hold light hand weights (1/2 – 3 lbs) or water bottles in each hand, sides of the hands touching each other. ■As you bend your knees to plie, zip the arms up the front of the body. ■ Let your elbows pop out wide. ■As the knees, straighten, zip the arms down the front of the body.

■Try this move with the **tops of the hands** touching each other. ■Try this move with your **palms facing** each other as well. ■Doing this exercise with three different hand positions creates a stronger, shapelier arm.

For each movement: try 5x today, work up to 10x

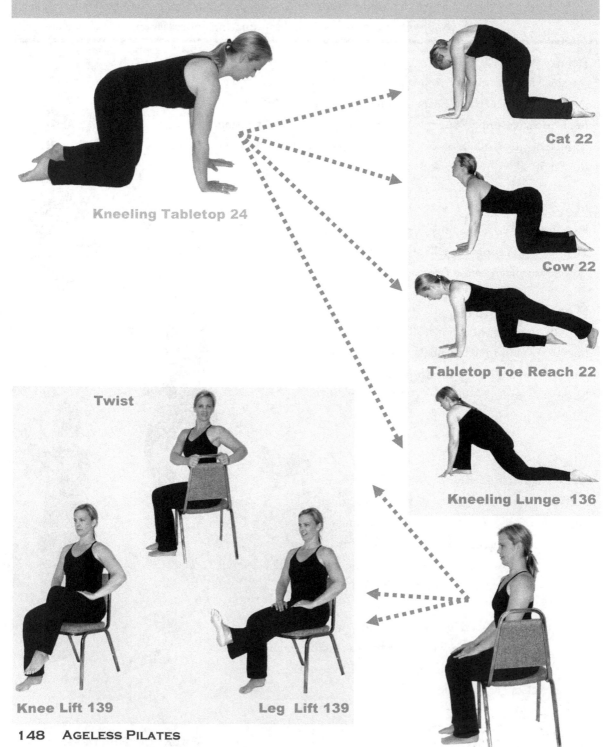

WORKOUT 10: BUILDING BALANCE

Kneeling Tabletop 24

Cat 22

Cow 22

Tabletop Toe Reach 22

Kneeling Lunge 136

Twist

Knee Lift 139

Leg Lift 139

Perform each movement group 5x, before moving to the next group.
Work up to 10x Use the page numbers for instructions & anchor points.

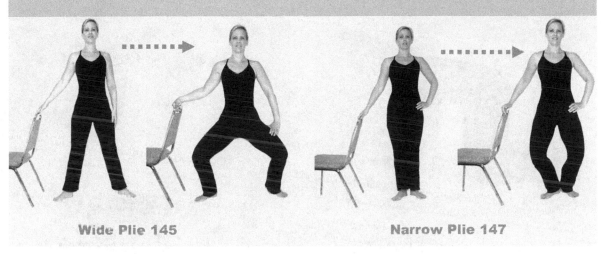

Wide Plie 145

Narrow Plie 147

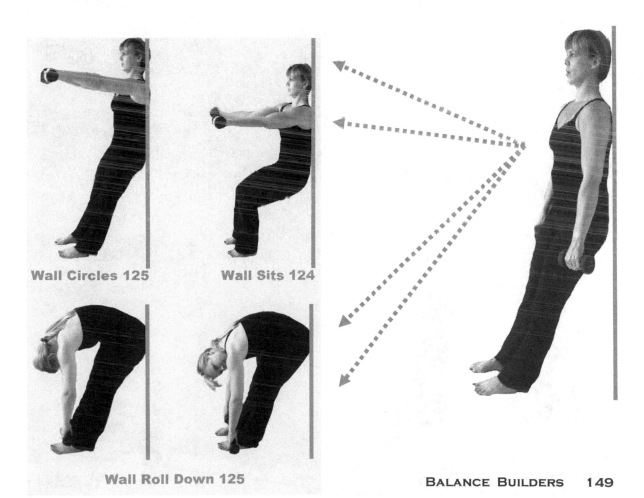

Wall Circles 125

Wall Sits 124

Wall Roll Down 125

WORKOUT 11: GROWING TALLER

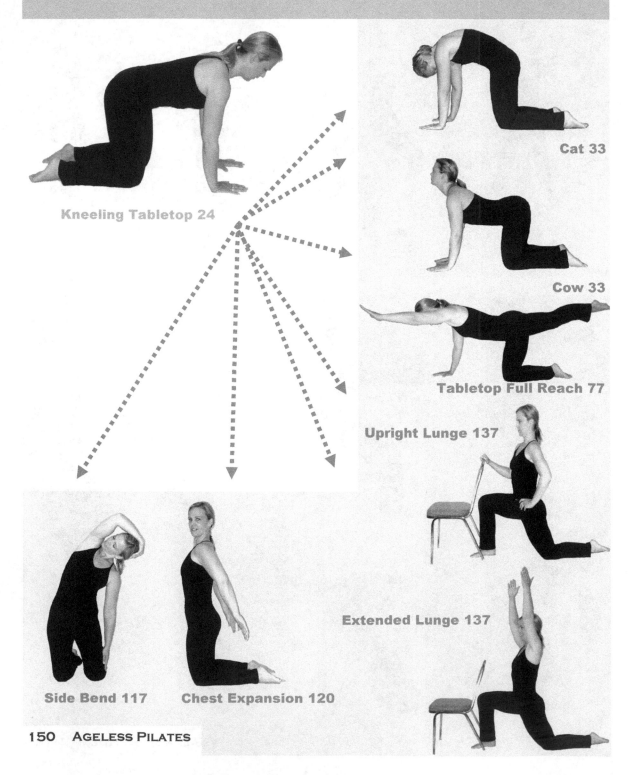

Kneeling Tabletop 24

Cat 33

Cow 33

Tabletop Full Reach 77

Upright Lunge 137

Extended Lunge 137

Side Bend 117

Chest Expansion 120

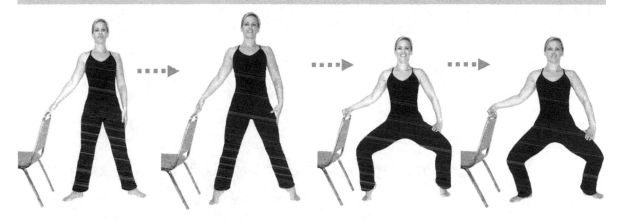

Wide Plie Heel Lifts 145

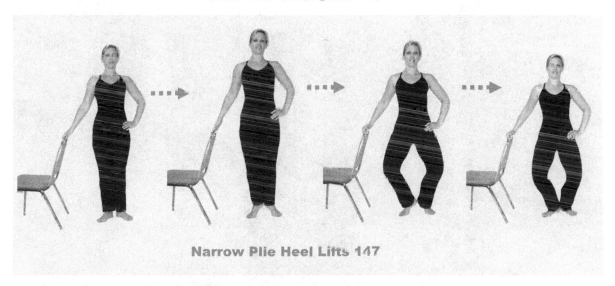

Narrow Plie Heel Lifts 147

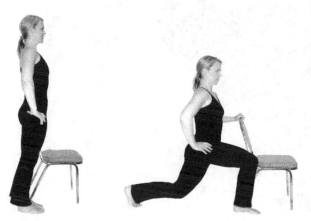

Forward Lunge 142

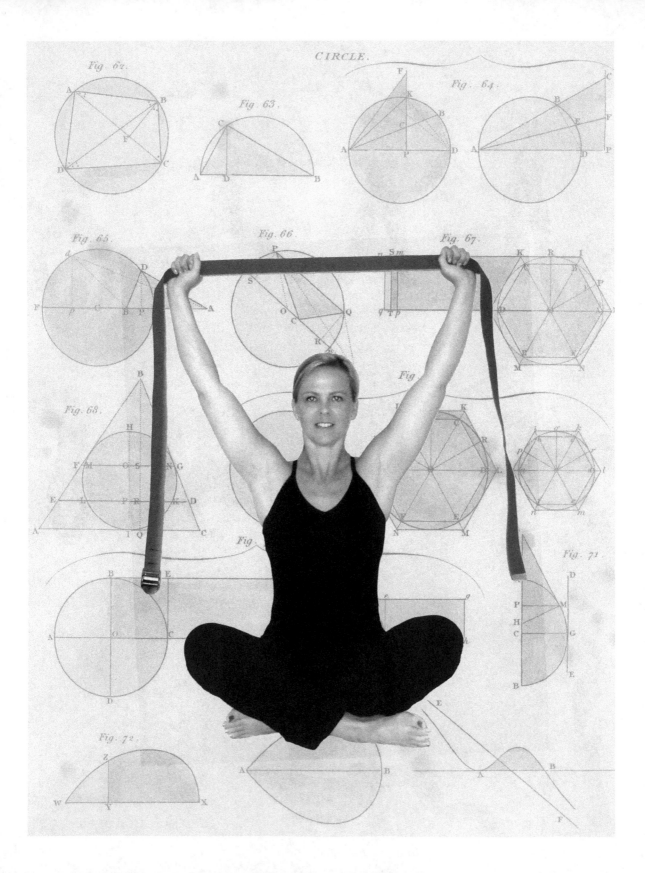

UPPER BODY MOBILITY

Do you remember when you could comfortably and easily turn and reach in all directions? When was the last time you did that? We all experience injuries small and large to our shoulder girdle, the area encompassing your collar bone, shoulder and shoulder blade. As those injuries heal, adhesions or knots form, leading to a smaller range of motion. The targeted movements in this chapter will work out those adhesions while stretching and strengthening the shoulder girdle.

Many report that these lessons have transformed their golf or tennis game by giving them back their youthful, easy upper body movements.

SHOULDER RANGE OF MOTION

The Range of Motion test engages your shoulders, chest and back while giving you an honest evaluation of the movement range you have available today. There is no need to push for a 'better grade,' simply move comfortably.

Anchor Points for this Lesson

- **Baseline;** scoop in from hipbone to hipbone.
- **Ribcage;** knit the ribs inward, as if you were wearing a corset.
- **Seat;** squeeze your bottom.

In all positions
- Lengthen toward both the ground and the sky.

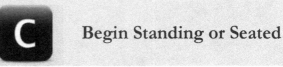
Begin Standing or Seated

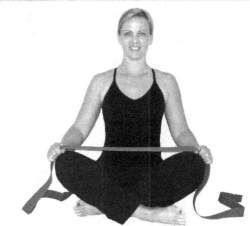

Whether you are standing or seated, scoop up the kittens, lengthen your spine and squeeze your seat.

Illegal Movement Alert!
Always move in a range of motion that does not cause pain

This means that your movement may be much smaller than the one I'm showing on the right. Your arms may not lift all the way, and they may not drop back. That's ok!

Working through pain can create a **compensation pattern.** This is when other muscles work to compensate for the painful area, setting you up for over-use injuries.

If you are experiencing an **arthritis** or **bursitis** flare-up, proceed with caution. Do not lift your shoulder into the range that causes pain. Doing so will increase, not help your pain.

TRY THIS RANGE OF MOTION TEST BEFORE & AFTER THE EXERCISES IN THIS CHAPTER

Begin in **Standing or Seated Neutral** position, holding the ends of a strap or towel in each hand. Inhale to prepare for the movement.

■While melting your shoulders down, float the arms up. ■Notice that I have plenty of space between my shoulder and ear in the photo.■If your shoulder raises up, then you've lifted your arm too high.

■Very gently rotate your arms backward to see how far you can comfortably bring your arms back. ■**Do not force this movement at all.**

■Note how far you can rotate the arms back ~ Just a little past your head? ~ To your ear? ~All the way to your backside? ■Does one arm move more comfortably than the other? ■**Notice:** how far apart do you need to hold the ends of the strap or towel?

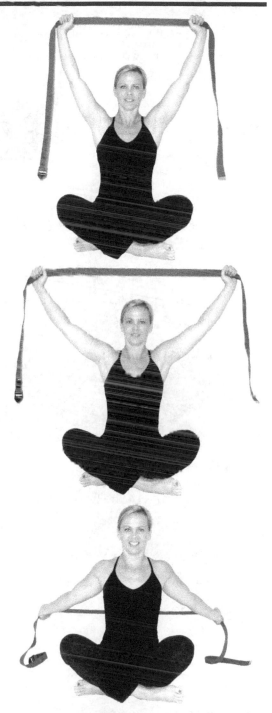

LESSON 23: MOBILE SHOULDERS

The Mobile Shoulders Lesson lubricates the joints and sends blood coursing through your shoulder muscles. This one-two punch increases your range of motion, allowing you to move your arms, neck and head with ease.

Begin Standing or Seated

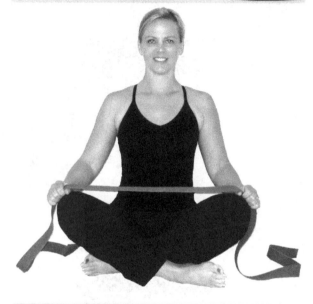

Do all of these Movements

- **W-Drops & 1-arm W-Drops**
- **Chest Pulls & 1-arm Chest Pulls**
- **Steering Wheel**

Anchor Points for this Lesson

- **Baseline;** scoop in from hipbone to hipbone.
- **Ribcage;** knit the ribs inward, as if you were wearing a corset.
- **Seat;** squeeze your bottom.

In all positions
- Lengthen toward both the ground and the sky.

Body Geometry

Tip: Sit or Stand in a Dignified Manner

While keeping your muscles comfortably engaged, create space between your ear and shoulder. Now create space between your ribs and hips. Being tense doesn't help the body, but being dignified in your posture does help in maintaining **Proper Body Geometry**.

A	B	C
W-Drops	**Chest Pulls**	**Steering Wheel**

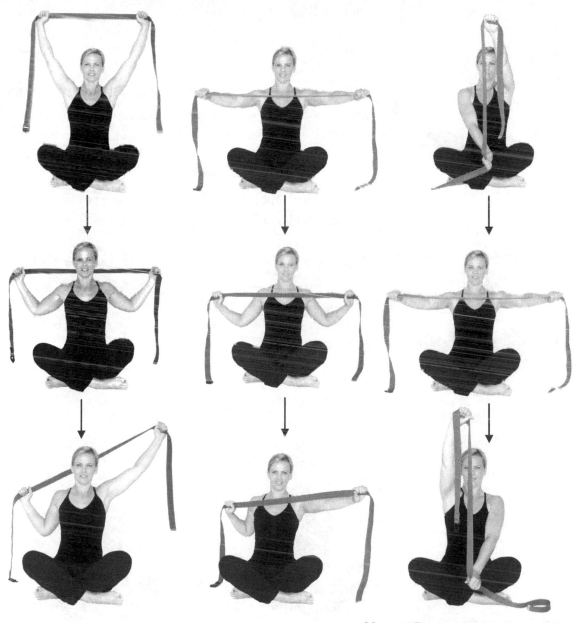

W-DROPS

W-Drops stretch your chest, strengthen your back, and help shift a rounded shoulder posture into a more open stance.

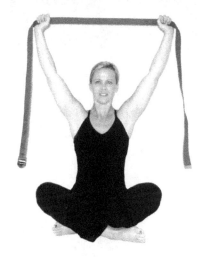

Begin in **Standing or Seated Neutral** position, holding the ends of a strap or towel in each hand. **Float your arms upward,** keeping your armpits low.

Inhale to prepare for the movement.

■Exhale as you lower just your elbows, as far as you can without any strain. Slide the towel behind your head. ■From the front, you will look like the letter W. ■Notice where your body feels a stretch. ■Inhale as you float the towel above your head again.

■Exhale as you lower the towel in front of your head in the W position. ■**Notice** where your body feels a stretch.

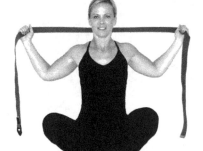

Repeat 5x times behind your head, 5x in front of your head.

■**Notice** where your stuck spots are; can you easily even out your movement when you become aware that there is a compensation pattern?

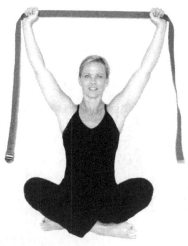
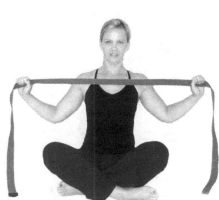

You'll become aware of comfort differences when you switch your movement to only one side at a time. Awareness is the first step in coaching your body toward positive change.

Begin in **Standing or Seated Neutral** position, holding the ends of a strap or towel in each hand. **Float your arms upward**, keeping your armpits low.

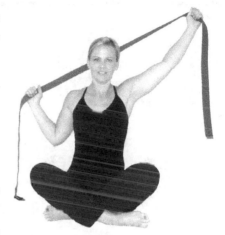

Inhale to prepare for the movement.

One-arm W drops

■As you exhale, lower only one elbow behind your head. ■ Inhale to bring the strap above your head again. ■Alternate from side to side. ■Notice where your body feels a stretch. ■Notice whether you can lower one elbow further than the other. As you continue to practice, this will likely balance out over time.

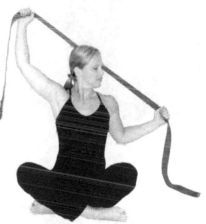

■Now try lowering one elbow at a time in front of your head. Can you lower one elbow further than the other? ■ Notice where the stretch has shifted to.

One-arm W drops with head turns:
■As you perform 1-arm W drops, **turn your head to the side with the lowered elbow**. ■Alternate from side to side, noting whether it is more comfortable to turn your head to one side than the other.

■Now **try turning your head to the opposite side** from the lowered elbow. ■Is this more difficult for you?

CHEST PULLS

Chest Pulls energize you by drawing blood flow into your chest and back. You're working on the tiny muscle fibers that allow your shoulders to perform the greatest range of motion of any joint in your body.

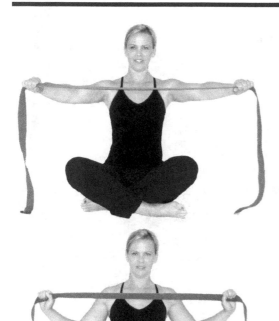

Begin in **Standing or Seated Neutral** position, holding the ends of a strap or towel in each hand. **Float your arms forward,** keeping your armpits low.

Inhale to prepare for the movement.

■Exhale as you bend your elbows, bringing the strap close to your chest. ■Tuck your elbows back comfortably. ■Notice where your body feels a stretch. ■Inhale as you return to your start position.

Repeat 5x

Next step: Try **One-arm Chest Pulls**

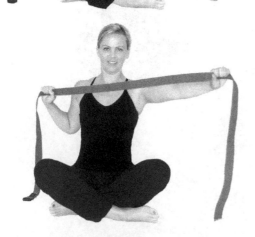

■As you exhale, pull only the right elbow back. ■Inhale to return to your start position. ■Alternate from one side to the next, noticing whether one arm moves differently than the other. This will likely balance out over time.

Repeat 5x to each side.

STEERING WHEEL

Steering Wheel stretches the muscle fibers around your shoulder blades. This is helpful for athletes who want to increase their arm movement speed, as well as for everyday people who want to scratch their own back 📑

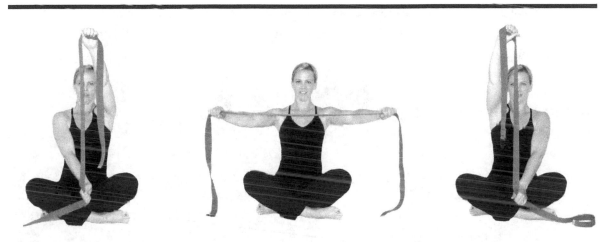

Begin in **Standing or Seated Neutral** position, holding the ends of a strap or towel in each hand. **Float your arms forward,** keeping your armpits low. Inhale to prepare for the movement.

■Exhale, as you lift your right arm high and your left arm low. Envision that you are steering the wheel on a ship. ■Keep your armpits low. ■Notice where your body feels a stretch. ■Inhale to return to your start position.

■Exhale, as you lift your left arm high and your right arm low. ■Inhale to return to your start position.

Repeat 5x to each side.

Body Geometry Tip: These Movement Patterns are wonderful for Building Brain Power

Learning movements that require a new type of coordination forces your brain to build new communication pathways. Why do we need these? Every day, millions of our brain cells die off. This is a normal part of being human. When we have many communication pathways in the brain, losing a few each day doesn't affect us very much,

Having many options, and the ability to build more, keeps your brain youthful.

LESSON 24: SECRET WEAPON

The Secret Weapon Lesson strengthens the deep abdominal muscles that criss-cross your body. To do this, you'll add spinal rotation to your shoulder movements. Learning to move your ribs separately from your hips creates a stronger, more powerful core. Your body uses this power in golf, tennis, running and walking.

Begin Standing or Seated

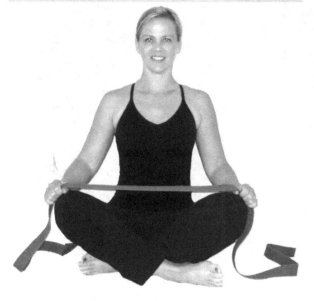

Anchor Points for this Lesson

- **Baseline;** scoop in from hipbone to hipbone.
- **Ribcage;** knit the ribs inward, as if you were wearing a corset.
- **Seat;** squeeze your bottom.

In all positions
- Lengthen toward both the ground and the sky.

Perform all of these Movements

- **Spine Twist**
- **Drawing the Bow**
- **Canoeing**

Body Geometry Tip:
Orient your Navel Forward

Whether you are seated or standing, keep your belly button pointed forward as your ribcage rotates. This creates a stronger core that will give you more flexibility in your daily life.

A	B	C
Spine Twist	**Drawing the Bow**	**Canoeing**

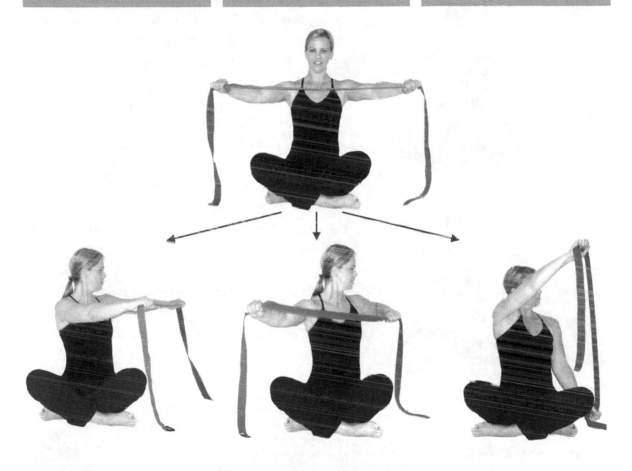

Rotate with Both Arms Straight	Rotate with Back Elbow Bent	Rotate with One Arm Up Other Arm Down

SPINE TWIST

Twists create a rejuvenating effect on the spine by opening up pockets of space for your discs and by freeing up constrictions on the spinal nerves. Always move gently during a twist as it is also possible to compress a nerve -- if you feel any discomfort, stop and gently reverse your movement.

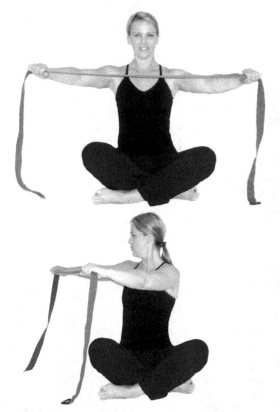

Begin in **Standing or Seated Neutral** position, holding the ends of a strap or towel in each hand. **Float your arms forward,** keeping your armpits low. ■Inhale to prepare for the movement.

■Exhale as you rotate your ribcage to the right. ■ Keep your hips still and quiet. When performed standing, this is more difficult than it sounds! ■ Inhale to return to your start position.

■Exhale as you rotate to the left, keeping the hips quiet. ■**Notice** how the stretch has moved to the muscles connecting the ribcage to the hips.

■Notice whether you can rotate more to one side than the other. Know that your range of motion will improve as you continue to practice this movement.

Repeat 5x to each side.

Comfort Option: What's your Range of Motion?

■When you first try this exercise, note how far you can see over your shoulder and ear.
Re-check this occasionally. This range of motion will increase quickly. ■If you've lost your ability to turn to see your blind spot when driving, this ability may return.

DRAWING THE BOW & CANOEING

See if you can feel the small muscle fibers around your shoulder blade stretch and release a bit more in this enhanced movement pattern

Begin in **Standing or Seated Neutral** position, holding the ends of a strap or towel in each hand. **Float your arms forward,** keeping your armpits low.

Inhale to prepare for the movement.

■Exhale as your rotate the ribcage to the right **and** pull your right elbow back. Leave your left arm extended straight. ■Keep the hips oriented forward, allowing your head to follow your moving elbow. ■ **Notice** where your body feels a stretch. ■Inhale to return to your start position.

■Alternate moving from one side to the other, noting if the movement is easier to one side.

Repeat 5x to each side.

■**Next Step**....try turning your head to the opposite side. This is more difficult than it would seem!

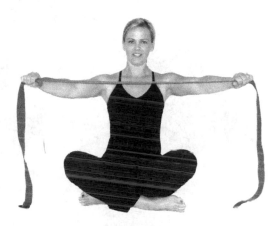

Back elbow is bent

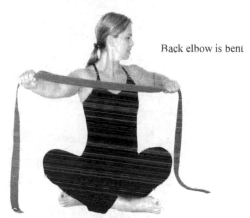

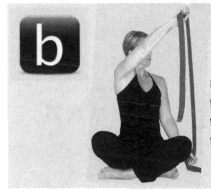

Body Geometry Boost:
Try Canoeing

■As you exhale and lift your right arm high, rotate your ribcage to the left. Keep your navel pointed forward. Let your head turn to look over your shoulder. ■Inhale to return to your start position. ■Exhale as you switch sides. ■Repeat 5x to each side.

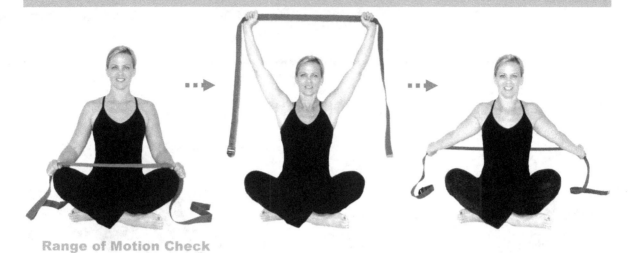

Range of Motion Check

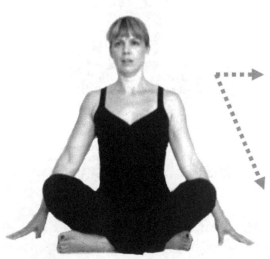

Seated/Cross Leg 23

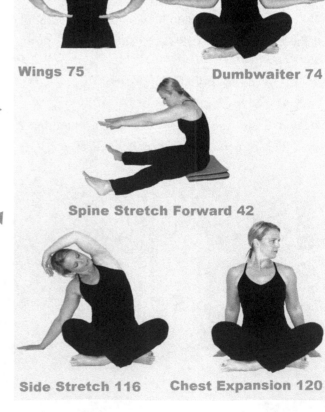

Wings 75

Dumbwaiter 74

Spine Stretch Forward 42

Side Stretch 116

Chest Expansion 120

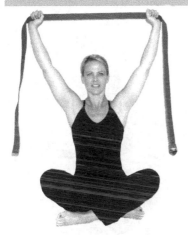

Seated/Cross Leg 23

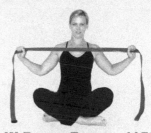

W-Drops Forward158

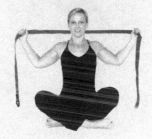

W-Drops Backward158

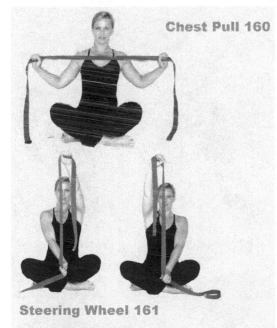

Chest Pull 160

Steering Wheel 161

Spine Twist 164

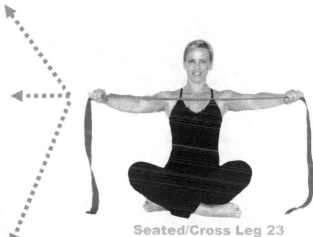

Seated/Cross Leg 23

Repeat Range Of Motion Test, never
forcing the movement.
Small changes over time will add up!

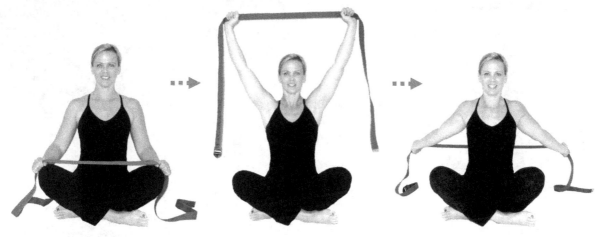

Range of Motion Check 165

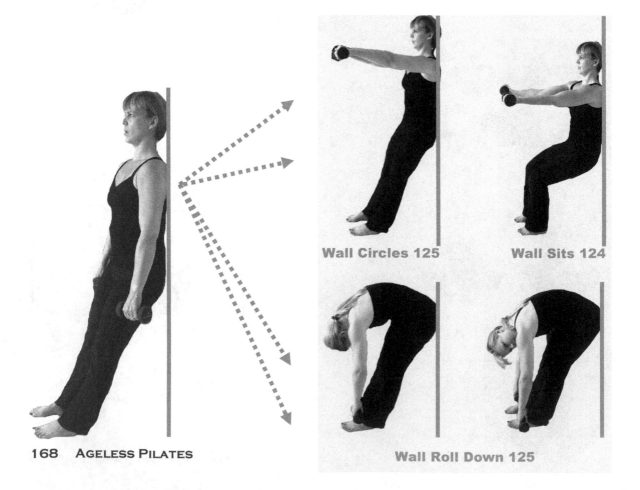

Wall Circles 125

Wall Sits 124

Wall Roll Down 125

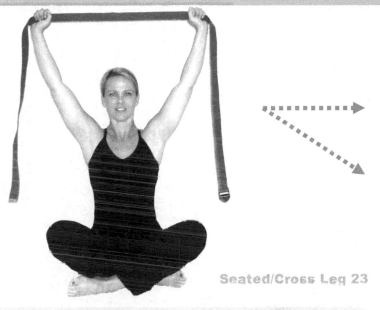

Seated/Cross Leg 23

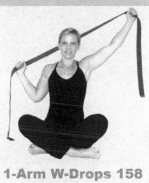

1-Arm W-Drops 158

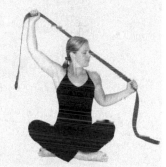

W-Drops with Head Turn 158

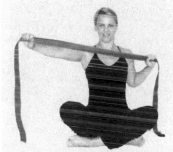

1-Arm Chest Pull 160

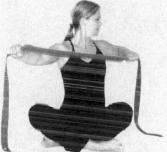

Drawing the Bow 165

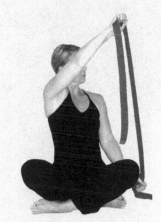

Canoeing 165

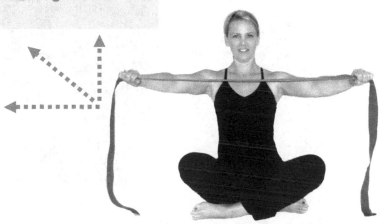

UPPER BODY MOBILITY   169

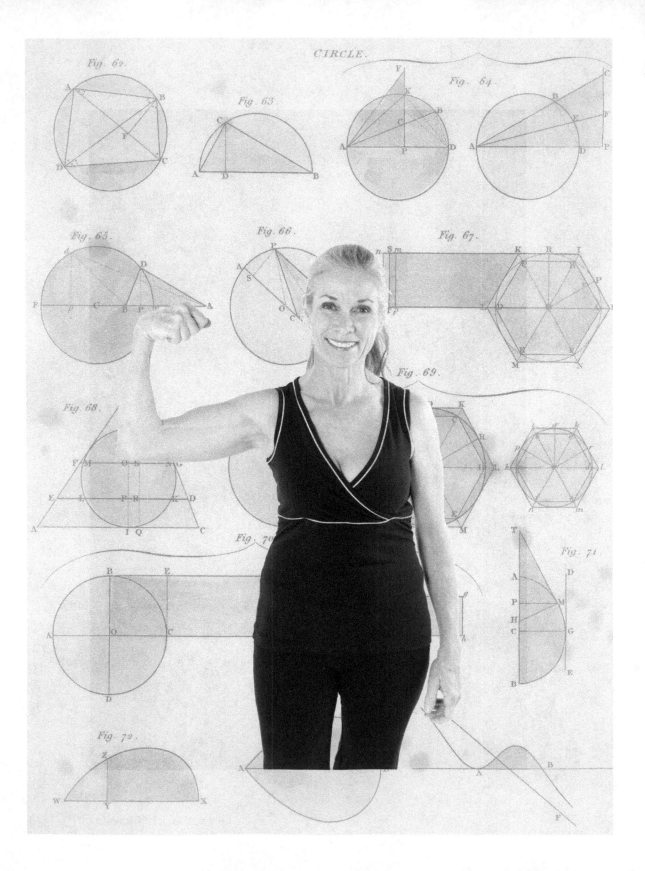

CIRCLE.

Fig. 62.

Fig. 63.

Fig. 64.

Fig. 65.

Fig. 66.

Fig. 67.

Fig. 68.

Fig. 69.

Fig. 70.

Fig. 71.

Fig. 72.

8

WORKOUTS
FOR
AILMENTS

Thousands of people, from all walks of life, have benefited from the Ageless Pilates system. If you have pain today, or are suffering from a loss of mobility, take heart. **You can improve the way you feel. You can increase your comfort when moving!**

It is reasonable to bring this book in to your health care provider to get an expert opinion on which exercises are best for your specific condition. Listen to your body. Keep your movements small at first, and always stay within your comfort range. Move a little bit everyday. On the bad days, keep moving, but give yourself a bit of leeway to make your movements smaller and fewer. On the good days, move a little bit more and a little bit bigger. Those little bits will add up to big change.

Low Back Pain is one of the

most common ailments in the United States. Nearly 50% of adults report that they have experienced pain in this area that has lasted more than 24 hours, at some point in the last year. If misery loves company, low back sufferers have literally millions of cohorts.

Common causes of back pain:

- **Muscular Strains**— maybe you moved in a way that your back did not appreciate, like hoisting a piano. Or perhaps longtime misalignment habits, like sitting in a slouched position, have finally caught up with you.

- **Herniated Discs & Compressed Nerves**— something within your body, a disc or a misaligned joint, is pressing inappropriately on a nerve,

- **Osteoporosis**— low bone density may have led to collapsed vertebra. Even a tiny amount of bone loss can be painful, as your body needs its natural support structure, your skeleton.

- **Fibromyalgia**—chronic muscle fatigue is the hallmark of this disease, which can leave sufferers with ongoing low-energy as well.

The Ageless Pilates system can help

- **Use the Repositioning pose and Stretches to Calm a Cranky Low-back.** These gentle movements help you place the bones and muscles of your pelvis and low-back in their best Body Geometry. Use these individually or as a group to stop painful muscle spasms, or to maintain a comfortable low-back.

- **Use the gentle Strengthening Moves to create a body that is able to hold itself with proper Body Geometry**. These movements will train the muscles around your pelvis to position you properly for daily life. **Do Pelvic Tilt for 60 seconds and Toe Taps for 120 seconds.** Slow and precise is better than quick and sloppy, so take your time and listen to your body.

Ongoing Backcare Lessons
- **Spine Warm-up** p.30
- **Leg & Hip Moves** p.58
- **Balancing Abdominals** p.66
- **Lower Ab Focus** p.90
- **Working the Wall** p.122

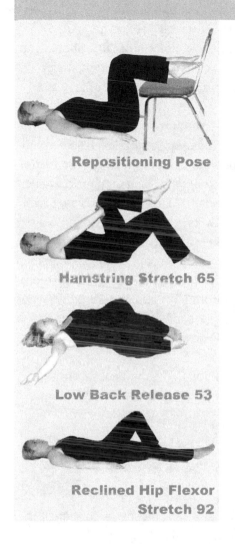

Repositioning Pose

Hamstring Stretch 65

Low Back Release 53

Reclined Hip Flexor
Stretch 92

Repositioning Pose

■Place your calves on a sturdy piece of furniture, entirely releasing the weight of your legs. ■Arrange your thighs perpendicular to the floor, not on an angle. Your hip should make a right angle, and your knee should make another right angle. ■Lay comfortably like this for at least 5 minutes.

Repositioning Stretches

■These three moves will allow your pelvis to re-set to its proper position. ■If it's more comfortable, you can perform the Reclined Hip Flexor Stretch with one leg propped up as in the Repositioning Pose. ■Use a large pillow to keep the toes of your extended pointed toward the sky. ■You should feel this stretch near your front hip bone.

Gentle Strengthening Moves for your Low-Back
■Try Pelvic Tilt and Toe Taps **with your hips on a rolled up towel** or a small, comfortable ball.
■Place the prop higher than your tailbone and lower than your waistband. This position should feel surprisingly comfortable. It will increase your range of motion, allowing you to gently release tight muscles.

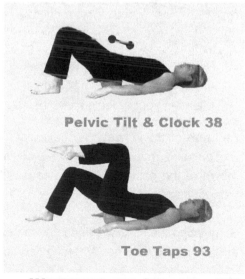

Pelvic Tilt & Clock 38

Toe Taps 93

Arthritis
affects more than 43 million people in the United States. Fifty percent of those over age 65 live with some type of arthritis, yet the majority of those living with the disease are even younger.

Osteo-arthritis (OA) is the most common type, involving the deterioration of joint cartilage. As the cartilage breaks down, joint movement can feel rough and painful in the hands, spine, knees or hips.

Rheumatoid arthritis (RA) involves the inflammation of the joint lining, also called the synovial membrane. This inflammation is often felt throughout the entire body, so it can feel flu-like. Joints swell and feel puffy or heated to the touch. Enzymes within the swollen areas eat away the cartilage, and can eventually deteriorate the bone itself.

Intelligent Exercise Can Ease Arthritis Pain

Although there currently is no cure for Arthritis, research has found that moderate exercise can:

- ✔ Improve flexibility in your joints
- ✔ Increase your range of motion
- ✔ Maintain your muscle strength

All three of these areas — flexibility, range of motion, and muscle strength — will help you minimize the pain that is often caused by both categories of arthritis.

Stimulating the cartilage in a joint can ease arthritis pain over time. When you compress a joint with exercise, fluids and toxins are flushed out. Release the compression, and fresh fluids packed with oxygen and nutrients seep in, creating healthier cartilage. This is particularly helpful for those with **signs of OA.** Should you have swollen or heated joints (symptoms of **RA**,) be moderate in your movements.

RA sufferers often report feeling more muscle stiffness and edema (generalized fluid retention) after periods of inactivity. Ageless Pilates can help you keep your joints mobile and flush out pooled fluids. A little bit of intelligent exercise once or twice a day can go a long way in maintaining full mobility and lessening joint pain. Let your body be your guide; if the pain is lessening with movement, it's ok to do more! Take advice from your health care provider for tips on treating the inflammation itself, as this is what will break down the joint over time.

All of the Ageless Pilates exercises are appropriate for those managing arthritis symptoms.

Comfort Options:
Honor what your body is telling you

Pain can be a tricky message to translate when you have arthritis.

■Be conservative in your choice of **position** and **range of motion**. ■Evaluate how you feel after 5 repetitions. ■Some people find that moderate amounts of movement are perfect for them, some need less. Some feel best with lots of movement.

Lessons that are particularly helpful in Easing Arthritis Pain

Spine
- **Spine Warm up** p. 32
- **Lengthen the Spine** p.7 8
- **Side Stretch** p. 114
- **Chest Expansion** p .118

Hip
- **Leg and Hip Warm up** p. 48
- **Leg & Hip Moves for Stretch** p .60
- **Kneeling Lunge** p. 36
- **Standing Balance** p. 138
- **Standing Lunge** p. 140

Knee
- **Seated Leg Work** p.169

Shoulder
- **Shoulder Warm up** p. 44
- **Shoulder Placement** p .73
- **Seated Arm Work** p.168

Add these Movements to maintain mobility in the Hands and Feet

Hands
If a hand, wrist or finger is more stiff, it is ok to use your other hand to assist the movement. Don't force yourself into any range that causes more pain.

- **Circles:** rotate your hand at the wrist 5x in one direction, and 5x in the other direction. Now try the other hand.

- **Wrist flex & flop**: gently draw the top of your hand back toward your wrist, then flop it in the opposite direction. Repeat this 5x on each hand.

- **Castanets:** touch each finger individually to your thumb. Repeat this 5x on each hand.

  When this becomes easy, try touching each finger to the palm of your hand. Curl your fingers as much as possible.

- **Fist Flys:** make a firm fist, then open it wide, as if you were throwing rice at a wedding. Repeat this 5x on each hand.

Feet
- **Circles:** rotate your foot at the ankle 5x in one direction, and 5x in the other direction. Repeat this on your other foot.

- **Point & Flex:** gently draw your toes and foot toward your shin, then release. Repeat this 5x with both feet.

- **Monkey Feet:** sit a chair, and place a small hand towel on the floor just at your bare feet. Using one set of toes, grasp the edge of the towel and pull it toward you an inch or two. Alternate right foot, left foot; drawing the towel toward you until it is all balled up. Now push it away using your toes.

Low bone density, affects

more than 25 million people in the United States, primarily women.

Osteopenia is a condition where bone density is lower than normal. When bone density dips low enough to put you at a high risk of collapse or breakage, it is called **osteoporosis**. This condition often progresses painlessly until a bone breaks in the hip, spine or wrist.

Proactive Steps to Building Stronger Bones

✔ **Get your daily recommended amounts of calcium and vitamin D.** Your body needs these nutrients to build bones.

✔ **Avoid smoking and excessive alcohol.** These leech calcium from your bones, lowering their density.

✔ **Engage in regular weight-bearing exercise.** This stimulates bone growth. In children, this can mean longer bones. In adults, it means bone density.

What do they mean by weight bearing?

■According to ongoing studies at Oregon State University, the body needs 4-8x body weight impact to stimulate bones to increase their density. This is the equivalent of an adult jumping onto and off of an 8" step. ■**Swimming**, **walking**, and **bicycling**, while good for your body for other reasons, do not create this level of impact and **are not weight bearing exercises**.

■**A good rule of thumb:** muscle exertion paired with *impact*, or paired with *moving a weighted object* (lifting, carrying, pushing, pulling) builds bone density, while lung exertion builds a stronger heart and cardio-vascular system. ■**Weight bearing** exercises require you to focus on what you're doing to stay stable and in good form. You'll feel a large increase in the level of exertion in your *muscles*. Don't confuse this with huffing and puffing to catch your breath. ■**Many Pilates exercises** ask you to lift your body weight in a manner that will stimulate bone growth.

Caution: For those Managing an Osteoporosis Condition

This Bone Building section is intended for those who want to take steps to **prevent osteopenia and osteoporosis**. It is not intended for those who have been diagnosed with either of these conditions.

Although weight bearing exercise builds bone density, those who have been diagnosed with osteoporosis must take special care of their delicate bones. The stresses created by typical exercises may be too much for a bone with very low density, and you will likely have no warning before a fracture occurs. Do speak with your health care professional about what exercises would be appropriate for your personal needs. There are appropriate exercises for you! Seek out recommendations for your specific case.

This mini-workout puts stress on both the spine and the hips, creating denser bones in two of the most commonly fractured. Begin with no added weight, then add small water bottles, then work your way up using small hand weights. Listen to how your body feels! Add this to the Lessons below to build a complete Workout.

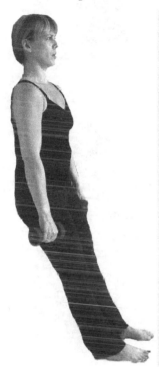
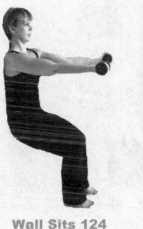
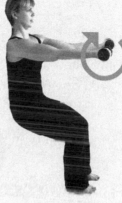
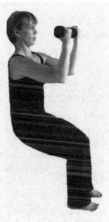

Wall Sits 124   **Add Straight-Arm Circles**   **Add Bicep Curls**

■Scoop up the Kittens and lengthen your spine. ■Slide your hips down the wall a bit. You don't need to come into a full sitting position at first, you simply need to feel your thighs working. ■Keep your knees pointed forward. This may be easier if you hold a small pillow or rolled up towel between them. ■Hold your Sit for 5 breaths, then stand up. ■Do Arm Circles 5x in each direction, then stand up. ■Do 5-10 Bicep Curls, then stand up.

Lessons that Build Bone Density in the Hip:
- **Working the Wall** p.122
- **Lengthen and Strengthen** p.130
- **Feeling Tall** p.132
- **Standing Balance** p.138
- **Standing Lunge** p.140
- **Standing Wide Plie** p.144
- **Standing Narrow Plie** p.146
- **Building Balance** p.148
- **Growing Taller** p.150

Lessons that Build Bone Density in the Spine:
- **Tabletop Reach** p.76
- **Lengthen the Spine** p.78
- **Matwork Basics** p.82
- **Long & Strong** p.84
- **Spine Extension** p.126

Stroke, diabetes, joint replacement surgery

and many other causes can all leave you temporarily or permanently chair-bound. Exercise is still important for your well being. It improves mood and metabolism, as well as boosting your ability to use your body to its fullest potential.

▪Perform each movement 5-10x

▪Try the arm movements with or without small hand weights. Make each movement small and precise at first. Add a larger range of motion as you become more comfortable.

Also Try:
▪**Mobile Shoulders** p.166
▪**Secret Weapon** p.168

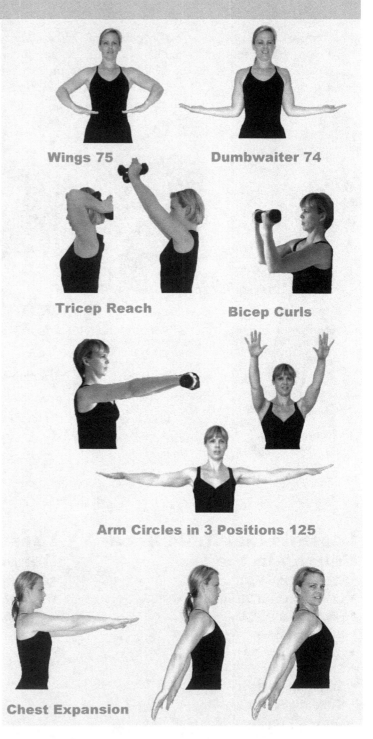

Wings 75

Dumbwaiter 74

Tricep Reach

Bicep Curls

Arm Circles in 3 Positions 125

Chest Expansion

MINI-WORKOUT 18: SEATED LEG WORK

There are times when re-learning to lift a leg is hard work! Try looping a strap around the leg or foot. You can use your arms to assist the movement.

Remember your Anchor Points: draw your armpits toward your hips.

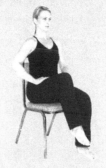

Knee Lifts 148

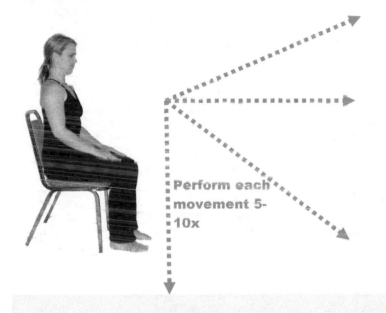

Perform each movement 5-10x

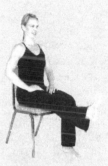

Leg Extend 148

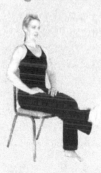

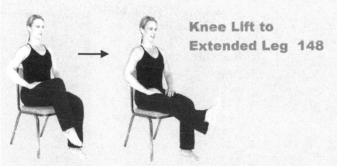

Knee Lift to Extended Leg 148

Add these movements:

- Tiny Leg Circles in both directions

- Foot Flexes

- Foot Circles in both directions

INDEX

Anchor points 7, 9, 15-18, 21-22, 24-26, 30, 36, 42, 44, 48, 56, 60, 63, 66, 73, 76, 78, 86, 90, 95-96, 100, 104, 116, 118, 122, 126, 136, 138, 140, 146, 154, 156, 162

Arthritis 174-175
    Feet 175
    Hands 175
    Hip 48, 60, 36, 138, 140
    Knee 169
    Shoulder 44, 73, 168
    Spine 32, 78, 114, 118

Body Geometry 7, 13
    Balance your teacup 17   Baseline 14
    Center of movement 14
    Draw your box 16
    Place your shoulders 18
    Stack and Lengthen 19

Body Geometry Tips **14,** 16, 17, 23, 30, 32, 36, 39-41, 44, 46-47, 49-51, 53, 56, 60, 63-64, 68-69, 72-73, 75, 86, 90, 95, 99-100, 104, 117, 121, 124, 129, 137, 139, 142-143, 146, 156, 161-162, 165, 179

Bone Building 176-177
    Hip 122, 130, 132, 138,   140, 144, 146, 148, 150
    Spine 76, 78, 82, 84, 126, 177

Breath 9, 11, 30, 32, 73, 120-121

Comfort Options Comfort Options 7, **20,** 33, 35, 38, 43, 53, 62, 65-66, 74, 81, 94, 96, 98, 102-103, 107, 114, 118, 126, 138, 140, 144, 164, 174

Discs 17, 33, 40, 42, 65, **68,** 114, 164, 172

Exercises
    1-arm Chest Pulls 156,   **160,** 169
    1-arm W-Drops 156, **158,** 169
    50-50's **71,** 85
    Arm Circles **47,** 55, 57,   87
    Backward Lunge 140,**142**
    Bent Knee Roll Down 67, **70,** 87,111
    Bent Knee Roll Up 67, **71,** 87, 111

Bicep Curls **177**
Bridge **40,** 41, 82, 84, 87, 108
Canoeing 162, **165,** 169
Castanets **175**
Cat/Cow **33,** 54, 110, 132, 150
Chest Expansion 118, **120,** 130, 132, 150, 166, 178
Chest Expansion with Weights 118, **121**
Chest Pulls 156, **160,** 167
Childs Pose **35,** 83, 85, 110, 131, 133
Cobra 79, **80**
Cradle/Rocking Cradle 67, **68,** 83
Criss Cross 104, **107,** 111, 133
Cross Leg Side Stretch 114, **116,** 130, 166
Dart 79, **81,** 85
Dogtail **34,** 54, 110
Double Knee Drop 100, **102,** 108
Double Leg Stretch 96, **99,** 111
Double Straight Leg 100, **103**
Drawbridge 87
Drawbridge with weights 87
Drawing the Bow 162, **165,** 169
Dumbwaiter 73, **74,** 83-84, 130, 132, 166, 178
Extended Lunge 136, **137,** 150
Fencers Lunge **143**
Fist Flys **175**
Foot Circles **175**
Forward Lunge 140, **142,** 151
Hamstring Stretch b, 82, 173
Hand Circles **175**
Kegal **41**
Knee Drop & Drag **52,** 55
Knee Drops **51,** 55
Knee Lifts 138, **139,** 148
Knee Slides 90, **92**
Knee Stirs **62,** 82
Kneeling Lunge **136**
Kneeling Side Stretch 114, **117,** 132, 150
Leg Circles Strength **64,** 84, 111
Leg Circles Stretch **63,** 84
Leg Lifts 138, **139,** 148
Leg Slides **50,** 55, 57
Letter X 126, **129,** 131, 133
Low Back Release **53,** 55, 173
Lunging Arm Raises **142**

Narrow Plie 146, **147**, 149, 151
Narrow Plie Heel Lift 146, **147**, 151
Narrow Plie Zip Up 146, **147**, 151
Pelvic Clock **39**, 54, 82, 84, 108, 173
Pelvic Tilt **38**, 54, 82, 84, 108, 173
Point & Flex **175**
Pregnant Cat **32**, 54, 110
Puppet Arms **46**, 55
Reclined Hip Flexor Stretch **92**, 108, 17
Repositioning Pose **173**
Repositioning Stretches **173**
Ribcage Arms **47**, 55
Rolling Ball 67, **69**, 85
Runners Lunge Hip Flexor Stretch **93**, 111
Scoop up the Kittens **32**, 36
Seated Knee Lifts **148**, 179
Seated Leg Lifts **148, 179**
Shoulder Range of Motion 154, **155**, 166, 168
Simple Criss Cross 104, **106**, 109
Single Leg Raise 126, **128**, 131
Single Leg Stretch 90, **94**, 111, 133
Sphinx 79, **80**, 83, 85, 109
Spine Stretch Forward **42**, 54, 83, 85, 168
Spine Twist 162, **164**, 167
Starfish 56
Steering Wheel 156, **161**, 167
Straight Arm Circles **177**
Swimming 126, **129**, 133
Table Top Arm Circles 96, **98**, 108
TableTop Arm Reach 76, **77**, 82
TableTop Double Reach 76, **77**, 84, 110, 132, 150
TableTop Leg Reach 76, **77**
TableTop Toe Reach 76, **77**, 82
Toe Taps 90, **93**, 108, 173
Upright Lunge 136, **137**, 150
V Lunge 140, **143**
Wall Circles 122, **125**, 131, 149, 168, 178
Wall Rolldowns 122, **125**, 131, 149, 168
Wall Roll-up 67, **72**, 109
Wall Sits 122, **124**, 131, 149, 168, 177
W-drop with Head Turn **158**, 169
W-drops 156, **158**, 167
Wide Plie 144, **145**, 149, 151
Wide Plie Curl 144, **145**, 151
Wide Plie Heel Lift 144, **145**, 151
Wings 73, **75**, 83-84, 130, 132, 166, 178

Wrist Flex & Flop **175**

Feet 40-41, 144, 175

Fibromyalgia 172

Golden Rules 9

Illegal Movements 70-71, 76, 95, 106, 124, 128, 154

Joseph Pilates 7, 89

Jack Lalanne 7

Key Positions
    Kneeling Tabletop **24**, 30, 32-34, 54, 76-77, 82, 84, 110, 132, 136, 148, 150
    Kneeling Upright **24**, 75, 114, 117-118, 120-121, 132
    Mini Roll-up/Feet Flat **21**
    Mini Roll-up/Tucked **21**, 95-96, 98-99
    Pilates V **25**, 146
    Prone **26**, 78-81, 83, 85, 126, 131, 133
    Seated/Cross Legged **23**, 73-74, 114, 116, 130, 154-155, 158-169
    Seated/Knees Bent **22**, 66, 68-70, 83, 85, 111
    Seated/Legs Extended **22**, 42
    Standing **25**, 122, 124-125, 131, 138, 140
    Supine/Knees Bent **20**, 36, 38-40, 44, 46-48, 50-56, 60-65, 71-72, 82, 84, 90, 92, 104, 106-109, 130
    Supine/Legs Tabletop **20**, 93-94, 100, 102, 108, 111
    Wide Pilates V **25**, 144

Lessons
    Arm & Leg Coordination 96
    Balancing Abdominals 66
    Chest Expansion 118
    Corset Cinch 104
    Double Duty 100
    Kneeling Lunge 136
    Leg & Hip Moves 60
    Leg & Hip Warmup 48
    Lengthen the Spine 78
    Lower Ab Focus 90
    Mobile Shoulders 156

Narrow Plies 146
Pelvis Warm-up 36
Secret Weapon 162
Shoulder Placement 73
Shoulder Range of Motion 154
Shoulder Warm Up 44
Side Stretch 114
Spine Extension 126
Spine Warm-up 30
Standing Balance 138
Standing Lunge 140
Tabletop Reach 76
Wide Plies 144
Working the Wall 122

Easy Shoulders, Easy Neck 166
Feeling Tall 132
Growing Taller 150
Lengthen and Strengthen 130
Long & Strong 84
Low Back Tonic 173
Matwork Basics 82
Mobility Creates Strength 168
Seated Exercises 178-179
Starfish 56
Work the Powerhouse 110

Wrists 33, 175

Low Back Pain 76, 78, 81, 94, 96, 107, 126, 128, 172
-173

Low Bone Density 176

Lumbar Curve 17, 38, 102-103

Neck 44, 76, 95, 98, 102, 125

Osteo-arthritis 174

Osteoporosis 172, 176

Props 11, 33, 43, 62, 92, 140, 179

Range of motion 7, 9, 29, 33, 39, 47, 51, 53, 59-60,
63, 74, 81, 103, 107, 117-118, 120, 126, 142, 153-
156, 160, 164, 166-167, 173-174, 178

Romana Kryzanowska 7

Rheumatoid arthritis 174

Seated Exercises 46-47, 74-75, 116, 120, 125, 139,
155-166, 168, 178-179

Workouts
        Arthritis Relief 175
        Bone Building   177
        Build a Powerhouse   108
        Building Balance 148
        Building Blocks 54
        Drawbridge 86

Get More of the
AGELESS PILATES SYSTEM

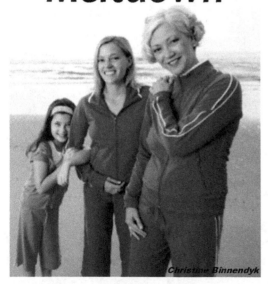

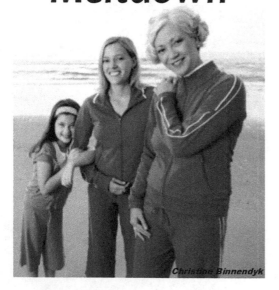

CPSIA information can be obtained
at www.ICGtesting.com
Printed in the USA
LVHW102330170919
631433LV00004B/57/P